Digestive Problems Solved

James H. Tabibian

Digestive Problems Solved

A Patient's Guide to Expert Insights
and Solutions

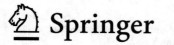 Springer

James H. Tabibian
David Geffen School of Medicine
University of California, Los Angeles
Los Angeles, CA, USA

ISBN 978-3-031-16319-7   ISBN 978-3-031-16317-3   (eBook)
https://doi.org/10.1007/978-3-031-16317-3

This Springer imprint is published by the registered company Springer Nature Switzerland AG
The registered company address is: Gewerbestrasse 11, 6330 Cham, Switzerland

Foreword

Reading Dr. Tabibian's fabulous book reminded me of the first time I saw the movie "Fantastic Voyage," an adventure where a team of scientists and a submarine, the Proteus, are miniaturized and injected into a man's body to repair a blood clot in his brain. We join the crew as they travel through the bloodstream, lungs, and small intestines and are even attacked by white blood cells. *Digestive Problems Solved* takes us on a real trek through the digestive system and the myriad problems that can arise (did you know that a dentist could recommend a consult with a gastroenterologist?). Dr. Tabibian knows his reader: we are not physicians who are well versed (or perhaps even all that interested) in esoteric medical jargon. Rather, we are people who need a comprehensive, easy-to-understand resource that will help essentially anyone improve their digestive health and, in turn, their quality of life. What sets *Digestive Problems Solved* apart is its focus on the whole person. Dr. Tabibian recognizes that there is no one-size-fits-all approach to digestive health and that factors such as stress, sleep, and exercise all play a role in how our bodies digest food and thus feel. By taking a holistic approach, he empowers readers to take control of their digestive health and improve their overall well-being.

Discussing digestive health means forthrightly tackling topics that some people find embarrassing. Dr. Tabibian jumps right in: we learn about hemorrhoids, dyssynergetic defection, fecal urgency, constipation, etc. with elegant yet clear explanations as to their etiologies, or what causes them. Just as importantly, he teaches us how to become better patients and self-advocates. We are provided tangible tools to elaborate on our ailments to enrich the provider-patient interaction ("The OLD CARTS" and "WILDA" symptom mnemonics await you!).

This book does not shy away from or disparage complementary and alternative medicine. It is indeed rare to find not just a gastroenterologist but a clinical professor at a premier research university with a Ph.D. enter the fray in such an open-minded, compassionate manner. We learn that Dr. Tabibian himself found relief with acupuncture at one point in his life. His humanistic vulnerability throughout forges a bond with the reader; we are not being harangued by an aloof expert but rather coached by a friend. We are, in a sense, in the aforementioned Proteus with him at the helm as he guides us on this extraordinary voyage.

I met Dr. Tabibian serendipitously on Twitter and was awed by his philosophy and positivity. While I am not a clinician, I have worked on the business side of healthcare for decades and frequently engage with thought leaders in this space in addition to also being in the final semester of my MPH program at Yale. I enthusiastically and unequivocally recommend *Digestive Problems Solved* as both a great primer on digestive health and a reference for when questions arise. It has a prominent place on my bookshelf, and I hope on yours as well.

To your good health!

Little Falls, NJ, USA   Jeffrey B. Benyacar Ed.D., MSc., MBA
February 2023

Preface

This book is a guide to understanding digestive problems, including what part of the gastrointestinal (GI) system they may affect, how often they occur, why they occur, what they may be an indicator of, how to evaluate them, what to do in terms of treatment, and how to generally stay well. It provides a foundation of core information, principles to reflect on, and tools to navigate your (or a loved one's or friend's) course with the countless potential digestive problems which may arise during our lives.

Why write this book? Well, at the age of 29, I underwent a surgery that unexpectedly changed my life...forever. Though much of the change was untoward, it ultimately made me a more empathic, careful, and attentive physician. In addition, looking back now close to a decade later on the health condition I had, I've realized how naïve and inadequately informed I was regarding the matter despite thinking that I had a solid grasp of the anatomy, my options, the process, and what to expect as far as surgical outcomes. So I thought to myself, if this was my experience as someone who already had years of medical education and training, how might non-medical professionals experience and navigate their way through their health problems and the healthcare system? Frankly, it's a bit of a scary (and lamentable) thought. Therefore, I came to feel a *bona fide* need to provide practical insights and direction for individuals who find themselves in the patient role, in particular those with digestive problems (given my subspecialty being in GI). The best and most far-reaching way I thought of doing so was through writing a book, and I felt a book of this nature was needed for many reasons. To name a few, so that our patients are less in the dark about their digestive health, to help demystify various aspects of medicine and healthcare, to equip patients with the know-how to more effectively interact with their healthcare providers and the healthcare system, and to aid them in being more enabled advocates.

In this book, I present insights and solutions that I've accrued and distilled based on years of schooling, training, practice, research, and teaching as well as my own history as a patient. Often times when a person has a digestive problem, it's not clear from the outset what it is, and even if it seems clear, there are certain ways of going about diagnosis and treatment that are comprehensive, principled in the fundamentals of medicine, and broadly applicable versus other ways that are not. This book will help buttress your health-related decision-making and steer you away from potential pitfalls in this regard and others. Depending on numerous factors, such as your education, experiences, digestive problems, diagnoses you've been given, treatments you've tried, and so forth, you might find certain chapters to be particularly enlightening and useful, whereas others may simply be a review or reinforce what you already know. If your familiarity in this arena is limited and you're like a clean slate per se, I believe you'll enjoy and benefit equally from the entire book. The mere fact that you've read it up to this point suggests that this book will address what you are hoping to find out or at least impart useful knowledge to help make you all the more informed with respect to digestive problems.

With in this book, I should mention from the outset that I use the expression "digestive problems," both liberally and inclusively. That is, by "digestive," I'm referring not only to digestion, but rather to the GI system overall. Similarly, by "problems," I am referring loosely to several and sometimes interchangeable terms, as shown here:

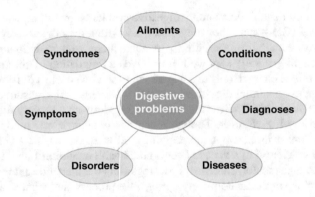

Illustration by Dr. Peerapol Wangrattanapranee, M.D.

Organizationally, you can expect the following in this book:

- Chapters are arranged in a logical chronological sequence and grouped into four sections, each with its own theme.
- Every chapter has a short introduction and is then broken up into headings and subheadings for ease of reading.
- I generally tried to keep things light and readily comprehensible wherever possible; at times, I opted to use medical terminology so that when you hear or come across it you aren't lost and so that you know it exists and can further read up on it.
- Figures and tables are included to illustrate, highlight, or expand upon certain points.
- At the end of each chapter, there is a "Putting it all together" section, wherein I've summarized the main points of the chapter.

I sincerely hope you enjoy this book and that it helps you overcome your digestive problems and preserve your digestive and overall health as well as that of your loved ones.

In solidarity, and with best wishes,

Los Angeles, CA, USA   James H. Tabibian

Acknowledgments

The process of writing, editing, and publishing a book is an undertaking that often requires the collective efforts of many people. Although I wouldn't be able to thank by name everyone who contributed to this process, I would like to herein specially express my gratitude to a few individuals. First, I thank all of the mentors, instructors, colleagues, friends, and patients who have made me a better physician, scientist, and/or writer; you've helped shape me into who I am today and equipped me with the tools necessary to conceive and complete this book. I also thank my Editor, Hannah Campeanu, for her keen feedback, encouragement, and guidance; in addition to making this book a reality, she elevated the quality and utility of my writing, both in this book and beyond. Lastly, and with all my heart, I thank my family; without my family, I would be nowhere and without direction.

Contents

Part I
The Gastrointestinal System and Digestive Problems: A Fundamental Primer

Chapter 1
Gastrointestinal Anatomy and Function: A High-Yield Overview

The anatomy and function of the human body can be organized into 10 major organ systems. The gastrointestinal (GI) system is one of these, as shown below:

- Cardiovascular (heart, arteries, veins, etc.)
- Endocrine (thyroid gland, adrenal glands, etc.)
- Gastrointestinal (esophagus, stomach, intestines, liver, etc.)
- Hematological (red blood cells, platelets, bone marrow, etc.)
- Immune (lymph nodes, tonsils, appendix, etc.)
- Integumentary (skin, hair, etc.)
- Musculoskeletal (skeletal muscles, bones, etc.)
- Nervous (brain, spinal cord, nerves)
- Respiratory (lungs, trachea, etc.)
- Urologic (kidneys, bladder, etc.)

The GI system is an extremely complex system of intricate parts and functions, and a healthy GI system is required for good health. Though the digestive tract, or the tubular portion, of the GI system comes to mind most readily, the GI system also encompasses other accessory organs and structures, including the liver, pancreas, gallbladder, and more. This chapter presents a brief, practical overview of the anatomy, and and physiology of the GI system, as relevant to common digestive problems.

© The Author(s), under exclusive license to Springer Nature
Switzerland AG 2023
J. H. Tabibian, *Digestive Problems Solved*,
https://doi.org/10.1007/978-3-031-16317-3_1

Anatomy of the GI System: What it Consists of

Digestive Tract

At the core of the GI system is the digestive tract, which spans from mouth to anus and largely occupies the abdomen (Fig. 1.1). The digestive tract goes by many names, including the alimentary tract, GI tract, and luminal GI system. It is an

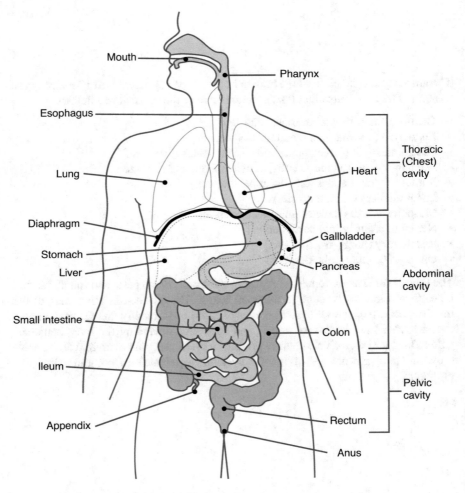

Fig. 1.1 Anatomy of the GI system: digestive tract and accessory organs and structures.
Legend: The digestive tract begins at the mouth and ends at the anus. It includes the esophagus, stomach, small intestine, and large intestine. The major accessory organs and structures of the GI system—the liver, gallbladder, and pancreas—are outlined with dotted lines; all three of these empty their digestive juices into the small intestine

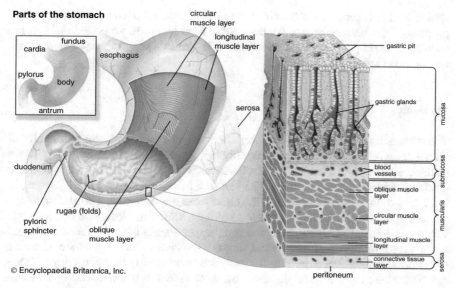

Fig. 1.2 Wall layers of the stomach as a representative organ of the digestive tract.
Legend: The organs of the digestive tract have multiple specialized wall layers: the mucosa (inner-most layer, lines the inside cavity, i.e. "lumen"), submucosa, muscularis, and serosa (outermost layer). Each of these layers has its respective components (e.g. glands, blood vessels, nerves) and functions, and there are unique adaptations and nuances from organ to organ. Notice, for instance, how the stomach has multiple sublayers of muscle, which fit its function as an organ that engages in rhythmic contractions (i.e. peristalsis) and mechanical churning of food to facilitate digestion

approximately 25-foot long tubular passageway through which food travels and is digested, absorbed, and ultimately expelled as waste. This passageway is formed by a series of four hollow, highly specialized organs that are in tandem with one another. Though hollow, these organs have complex wall structure, as shown in Fig. 1.2. Each organ generally has four essential wall layers: mucosa (innermost layer), submucosa, muscularis, and serosa (outermost layer).

Once food is received in the mouth, it is chewed, mixed with saliva, pushed back by the tongue, and then swallowed. These steps comprise what is known as "inges-tion". Because ingestion is initiated in the mouth, some would say that the mouth is actually the first structure of the digestive tract. Either way, once food is swallowed, it enters into the esophagus, the first of the four hollow organs of the digestive tract.

Esophagus

The esophagus, or "food pipe" as it's sometimes referred to, courses downward through the middle of the chest behind the heart and lungs and primarily serves to transfer food into the stomach. It is a 15–20″ long, straight tubular structure that is capped on either end by a sphincter, a ring-like muscular barrier. At the top portion of the esophagus, the upper esophageal sphincter (UES) separates it from the phar-ynx, or throat; at the bottom portion of the esophagus, the lower esophageal sphincter (LES) separates it from the stomach at a site referred to as the esophago-gastric (or gastroesophageal) junction. After food has been propelled through the esophagus and upon opening of the LES, it traverses through the esophagogastric junction and enters the stomach.

Stomach

The stomach is a large, bag-like muscular organ measuring approximately 12 inches long by 6 inches wide. It generally has a gentle curve to it at its mid-lower portion, similar to the letter "J" (or a backwards "C"), and has four main regions: cardia, fundus, body, and antrum. The stomach is located below the diaphragm, or breathing muscle, which separates the chest from the abdomen. The abdomen can be conceptually subdivided into four quadrants, which in clockwise fashion, are: left upper, left lower, right lower, and right upper. Parenthetically, these quadrants are a very common part of medical lingo, e.g. when describing where someone experiences abdominal pain. The stomach is located mainly in the left upper quadrant and where the left and right upper quadrants meet. It facilitates complex functions, as discussed in the next section, and has a sphincter at its distal end, or bottom portion, known as the "pylorus". Once the functions of the stomach have been completed (which may take 2–6 hours depending on the nature of the food ingested and other factors), the partially digested food and digestive juices, collectively referred to as "chyme", pass through the pylorus and into the small intestine.

Small Intestine

The small intestine, or small bowel, is the longest part of the digestive tract, approximately 15–20 feet in length. It is a winding structure that courses all over the abdomen, in all four quadrants. The small intestine is divided into three consecutive segments: duodenum, jejunum, and ileum (Fig. 1.3). Further digestion and eventual absorption take place in the small intestine, and each segment has its own nuanced features and functions. The last segment, the ileum, directly connects to the colon in the right lower quadrant of the abdomen through what is known as the ileocecal valve, yet another sphincter in the digestive tract. The total transit time of chyme through the small intestine is approximately 1–3 hours, depending on the food ingested as well as inter-individual variation.

Large Intestine

The large intestine, or colon, is the last organ of the digestive tract. It is approximately 4–6 feet in length and generally encircles the abdomen in a clockwise fashion, starting in the right lower quadrant of the abdominal cavity and ending at the rectum (which is in the pelvic cavity) and anus. Similar to the small intestine,

Fig. 1.3 Segments of the small intestine and large intestine.
Legend: The small intestine has three segments: the duodenum (first and shortest), jejunum (middle), and ileum (last and longest). The ileum drains into the colon, which itself has six segments: the cecum (to which the appendix connects), ascending colon, transverse colon, descending colon, sigmoid colon, and rectum

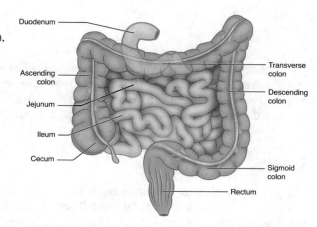

and as shown in Fig. 1.3, the large intestine is anatomically divided into segments: cecum, ascending colon, transverse colon, descending colon, sigmoid colon, and rectum. Connected to the cecum is the appendix, an approximately 4 cm-long, worm-shaped pouch. The rectum merges with the anus, through which food waste is eliminated from the body. The rectum and anus are surrounded by many structures that constitute the pelvic floor; these structures are directly or indirectly related to achieving effective elimination, also referred to as defecation or evacuation.

Accessory Organs and Structures

Along its long and windy course, the digestive tract receives different inputs or contributions from the accessory organs (as well as glands, nerves, blood vessels, etc.) and works synchronously with them. The three accessory organs are the liver, gallbladder, and pancreas.

Liver

The liver is a large, solid, fleshy organ located under the right rib cage in the right upper quadrant of the abdomen. It is home to extremely complex machinery critical to a numerous body functions, including filtering, processing, and refining food, beverage, and medication; storing energy from food that is digested and absorbed; and producing and releasing many different proteins and other substances. In the context of digestion, one of the key substances that the liver produces and contributes is bile, which is essential for digestion and subsequent absorption of lipids, or fats.

Gallbladder

The gallbladder is a small, bag-like structure located just below the liver in the right upper quadrant of the abdomen. It functions to store and concentrate bile that it receives from the liver through the bile duct system. In response to a meal, it releases bile into the duodenum by way of the common bile duct.

Pancreas

The pancreas is a slender, delicate organ located behind the stomach. It is shaped similar to a fish, with a head, body, and tail portion, and is roughly the size of one's fist. The pancreas' main role in digestion is producing and secreting digestive substances, including bicarbonate and enzymes such as amylase, lipase, trypsin, chymotrypsin, and elastase, into the duodenum. These are critical to further break down and process food that has entered the small intestine. The pancreas also has other functions, such as producing and secreting endocrine hormones (e.g. insulin) into the blood stream, which are critical to overall health.

Function of the GI System: How it Works

Now that we have discussed the physical parts of the GI system, let's talk about what they do. The GI system has many different roles in supporting the body as a whole. The primary overarching role of the GI system, in particular the digestive tract, is to receive, absorb, and prepare nutrients for utilization by other systems throughout the body and to rid the body of waste. This is achieved through concerted processes between the digestive tract and the accessory organs of the GI system. Overall, these processes can be organized into six main functions.

Six Main Functions of the GI System

Ingestion

As mentioned earlier in the chapter, ingestion refers to the process of eating: taking food in through the mouth, chewing it, moistening it with saliva, and swallowing it. Ingestion is the starting point for the remaining five functions.

Mechanical Digestion

Food that is ingested needs to be broken into smaller pieces. This is called mechanical digestion, and it occurs not only in the mouth (chewing) but also in the stomach, wherein churning and mixing actions occur.

Chemical Digestion

Facilitating mechanical digestion is chemical digestion, which includes the actions of saliva, digestive enzymes, gastric or stomach acid, and bile in helping to break down food. Interestingly, chemical digestion doesn't only begin when food is swallowed; it can be initiated by the mere sight, smell, thought, or taste of food, all of which comprise what is known as the cephalic phase of digestion. "Cephalic" comes from the Greek word for "head", which is to say that just having food on your mind can initiate the process. In fact, approximately 20% of gastric secretions associated with eating a meal occur during the cephalic phase.

Movements

The first major form or aspect of movement with regard to the digestive tract is ingestion. The swallowing portion of ingestion may seem simple, but is actually a highly regulated phenomenon that requires intricate coordination of muscles that are under control of the nervous system. Swallowing, also referred to technically as deglutition, is comprised of three stages:

– Oral: food being voluntarily moved from the mouth into the pharynx. This stage of swallowing is under volitional control because it involves skeletal rather than smooth muscle, which moves involuntarily.
– Pharyngeal: food being involuntarily transferred from the pharynx into the esophagus, generally only taking a second or two.
– Esophageal: food being involuntarily propelled through the esophagus to the stomach, generally requiring only 3–8 seconds.

These distinct stages require the concerted relaxation and contraction of various muscles so that food enters the proper place. For instance, if the UES does not relax when it's supposed to, food won't enter the esophagus upon swallowing and may instead go down into the lungs. With respect to the LES, if it does not relax when it's supposed to, food won't pass from the esophagus to the stomach, and conversely, if it relaxes at the wrong time, stomach contents can reflux back up into the esophagus.

The second form of movement in the digestive tract occurs in the stomach. Smooth muscle contractions serve to churn the food, expose food particles to digestive juices such as acid and enzymes, and break things down to a fine enough level for them to pass through the pylorus into the small intestine. As mentioned earlier, this partially digested food mixed with digestive juices is technically referred to as "chyme."

The third form of movement is an overarching one, spanning from the esophagus to the colon, and is what propels food particles through the digestive tract. It is known as "peristalsis", and it occurs in rhythmic waves of smooth muscle contractions.

Absorption

Absorption refers to the passage of molecules, or microscopic particles, of carbohydrates, fats, proteins, vitamins, and minerals through the membranes of the cells lining the small intestine. These nutrients ultimately make their way into the circulatory system and are carried to the liver for further processing. The small intestine has specialized absorptive functions, some unique to specific segments; for instance, iron is primarily absorbed in the duodenum, the first segment of the small intestine, whereas vitamin B12 is absorbed in the ileum, the third and last segment.

Elimination

The portions of food that cannot be digested or absorbed need to be eliminated from the body. Elimination of this waste material through the anus, in the form of feces, is known as defecation or evacuation. Though this may seem like a simple phenomenon, it requires synchronized coordination of the various muscles and other structures of the pelvic floor. At a high level, for normal evacuation to occur, the sphincter muscles of the anus must relax whilst the muscles of the pelvic floor and rectum contract, thus creating an outward pressure gradient. Lack of this normal function can result in "dyssynergic defection" or in "fecal incontinence," which are the main GI manifestations of a group of disorders under the umbrella of pelvic floor dysfunction.

Organic Versus Functional GI Disorders

An important distinction to make with digestive problems, and one relevant to the content of this chapter and book overall, is whether they are an "organic" vs. "functional" disorder. "Organic" disorders, in general, are those that are biochemically, morphologically, and/or anatomically detectable. "Organic" in this context is not the same as "organic" foods and has nothing to do with the absence of pesticides or hormones. An example of an organic disorder would be a gastric ulcer: it can be seen by endoscopy, among other means, as appearing different compared to normal stomach lining. Another example would be a rectal cancer: blood indices (or "biomarkers") suggesting cancer may be elevated, the cancer can be seen by colonoscopy and often CT scan, and biopsies of the cancer examined under a microscope can confirm the diagnosis. A third example of an organic disorder would be diabetes: it has fairly clear-cut biochemical markers in blood, such as fasting serum glucose and hemoglobin A1c. Organic disorders are also sometimes referred to as "structural" or "anatomical" disorders, but these terms only capture a subset of organic disorders; diabetes, for instance, isn't really a structural or anatomical disorder (though strictly speaking, some microscopic anomalies can indeed exist).

On the other hand, the term "functional" is used to describe a disorder that is biochemically, morphologically, and anatomically undetectable and thus not definable or diagnosable by these means. In other words, a functional disorder does not appear different than normal to the naked eye or by a CT scan, colonoscopy, or blood test, etc. Many times, the issue lies in how the body senses things or responds to a stimulus, but nobody really knows for sure, in part because there are many different functional disorders that can vary between individuals. Irritable bowel syndrome (IBS) is a hallmark functional disorder. The functional nature of IBS—namely the absence of detectable inflammation, mass, or other tell-tale signs—can often make accurate diagnosis challenging, sometimes leading to frustration for patients and providers and to unproductive comments such as, "It's all in your head." From my perspective, a functional disorder is as important to accurately diagnose and appropriately manage as an organic one.

Putting it all Together

In healthy, asymptomatic individuals, the anatomical and functional aspects of the GI system, including the digestive tract and the accessory digestive organs and structures, work properly behind the scenes to maintain digestive and overall health. When either of these aspects is disturbed, symptoms or signs of a digestive problem, whether organic or functional, may arise. When they arise, they may point to a number of different possible causes; some symptoms and signs are quite specific, meaning that they fairly clearly point to what and where the problem is, while many others are non-specific. This raises the need for patients and providers to work together to identify the possible causes, carefully investigate them, and hone in on the most likely one and in turn the most appropriate treatment. It is often tempting to use umbrella terms like "indigestion" or "gastritis," but these are often not really accurate nor helpful given they are vague, catch-all expressions.

With so many parts and functions, the GI system is truly something to marvel at, but at the same time breakdowns can and do occur. Just how common digestive problems are and the impact they have is covered next in Chap. 2.

Further Reading

https://www.kenhub.com/en/library/anatomy/stages-of-swallowing#:~:text=%20Swallowing%20
     is%20divided%20into%20three%20stages%3A%20,the%20esophagus%20and%20into%20
     the%20stomach%20More%20
https://www.ncbi.nlm.nih.gov/pmc/articles/PMC3831353/
Introduction to the digestive system. SEER Training (cancer.gov).
Phases of digestion. Boundless anatomy and physiology (lumenlearning.com).

Chapter 2
The Burden of Digestive Problems: Common and Impactful

A Disclaimer about Assessing the Burden of Digestive Problems

There are several challenges in accurately assessing how common digestive problems are. Posing the most difficulty in this regard is perhaps terminology. Terms like digestive, GI, gastroenterological, and gut have all been used in this space; sometimes they mean the same thing, but sometimes not. As alluded to above, terms such as ailment, condition, disorder, and disease are also all used. Depending on context, sometimes they are interchangeable, sometimes they are not, and many times they will be used interchangeably incorrectly! Have a look, for instance, at Tables 2.1 and 2.2, which provide lists of leading GI symptoms and physician diagnoses in the ambulatory and emergency department setting. As you can see, some terms are present in both lists; this is because they can be both a symptom (as reported by a patient) as well as a diagnosis (as determined by a provider). All in all, this variability in terminology creates a considerable number of permutations (e.g. digestive problem vs. GI symptom vs. gut condition vs….) and can make it difficult to present a clear and precise picture in terms of how common digestive problems are.

There are also a number of challenges in accurately assessing how *impactful* digestive problems are. Of course, some problems are clearly more impactful than others. Ironically, some problems which are not life threatening can be immensely bothersome and symptomatic, whereas others that are life threatening may have no symptoms. This clouds the picture in terms of how impactful digestive problems are all around. Similarly, it's difficult to quantify how common digestive problems are if some of them don't cause symptoms.

The original version of the chapter has been revised. A correction to this chapter can be found at https://doi.org/10.1007/978-3-031-16317-3_15

© The Author(s), under exclusive license to Springer Nature Switzerland AG 2023, corrected publication 2023
J. H. Tabibian, *Digestive Problems Solved*,
https://doi.org/10.1007/978-3-031-16317-3_2

Table 2.1 Leading gastrointestinal (GI) *symptoms* prompting a medical visit in the United States

Rank	Symptom	Estimated number of annual visits		
		Office	Emergency Department	Total
1	Abdominal pain	6,893,881	12,524,768	19,418,649
2	Vomiting	2,596,369	2,768,558	5,364,928
3	Nausea	1,636,346	2,304,775	3,941,121
4	Diarrhea	1,915,475	667,584	2,583,060
5	GI bleeding	659,135	874,612	1,533,747
6	Constipation	864,103	378,331	1,242,434
7	Anorectal symptoms	786,668	94,993	881,661
8	Heartburn/indigestion	680,031	43,432	723,463
9	Decreased appetite	511,705	59,662	571,367
10	Dysphagia	412,870	154,853	567,723
Total				36,828,153

Adapted from Peery et al. (Burden and Cost of Gastrointestinal, Liver, and Pancreatic Diseases in the United States: Update 2021–PubMed nih.gov))

Table 2.2 Leading gastrointestinal *diagnoses* prompting a medical visit in the United States

Rank	Diagnosis	Estimated number of annual visits		
		Office	Emergency Department	Total
1	Abdominal pain	7,979,815	7,693,205	15,673,020
2	Nausea and vomiting	2,569,377	2,469,273	5,038,650
3	GERD and reflux esophagitis	4,345,680	317,964	4,663,644
4	Constipation	2,226,455	854,399	3,080,854
5	Abdominal wall and inguinal hernia	2,468,048	289,434	2,757,482
6	Diarrhea	1,362,383	626,030	1,988,413
7	Hemorrhoids	1,803,032	86,514	1,889,546
8	Gastritis and dyspepsia	1,128,641	490,448	1,619,089
9	Cholelithiasis	863,398	326,985	1,190,383
10	Dysphagia	1,049,240	89,325	1,138,565
Total				39,039,646

Adapted from Peery et al. (Burden and Cost of Gastrointestinal, Liver, and Pancreatic Diseases in the United States: Update 2021–PubMed nih.gov))

Digestive Problems Are Common and Have a Profound Impact Nationally

There are some eye-opening statistics that should be noted with regard to digestive problems. For example, on an annual basis, in the United States (US) alone:

- Digestive problem symptoms account for over 36 million ambulatory visits. In other words, nearly 100,000 outpatient appointments take place daily because of symptoms of a possible digestive problem.

- There are over 43 million ambulatory visits with a primary diagnosis of a digestive problem.
- Hospitalizations for a digestive problem reach nearly four million, with over 400,000 readmissions.
- Healthcare expenditures for digestive problems total approximately 120 billion dollars.
- Nearly 300,000 new cases of digestive cancers are diagnosed.
- Digestive problems, including cancers, cause over 250,000 deaths.

These are compelling data that digestive problems are abound and consume an immense amount of healthcare resources. They are an important issue to healthcare professionals, policymakers, and taxpayers, and of course to those who suffer with them or are otherwise affected by them.

Burden OF Digestive Problems at the Individual Level

No matter how rare or common a digestive problem may be, if you're the one experiencing it, it's probably burdensome to at least some degree. How burdensome it is depends on a few things. First and foremost, it depends on its severity, or how bad the problem is, and its frequency, or how often it occurs. Moving beyond this, it also depends on how well you are able to cope with the issue physically and psychologically, which in turn depends on various factors, such as knowing whether or not:

- there is a safe and effective treatment for the problem
- the problem is expected to worsen
- it will last for a long time
- medications will be needed for life
- it can interfere with day-to-day life
- it may turn into cancer

For any given patient, these are questions that we, as providers, may know the answers to as part of our medical training. But for patients, these are often scary and unfamiliar topics that don't have obvious answers. Therefore, if you don't have the answer but wish to have it, by all means ask. You deserve to know; after all, it's your body. Of note though, for a considerable proportion of patients, we actually don't know the answer to many of these questions, and instead it's as though we are on a journey together to do the best with what we know and tackle together what may come in the future.

Putting it all Together

Digestive problems, whether they are ailments, disorders, symptoms, syndromes, or go by some other name, are very common and impactful in a number of senses. Sometimes they are just a minor nuisance or annoyance, whereas in other cases they can be life- altering or life-threatening. Interestingly, in some cases it's the non-life-threatening conditions that can seem to pose the most burden on one's quality of life, while life-threatening conditions can sometimes be initially insidious.

However common or impactful your digestive problem may be at a public health level, it's important to clarify how it relates to and affects you personally, do so early on, and determine if it may represent something that requires prompt healthcare professional evaluation. How to approach doing so is covered next in Chap. 3.

Further Reading

Burden and cost of gastrointestinal, liver, and pancreatic diseases in the United States: update 2021. PubMed (nih.gov).
Burden of digestive diseases in the United States report. NIDDK (nih.gov).
Gastrointestinal diseases: symptoms, treatment & causes (https://my.clevelandclinic.org/health/articles/7040-gastrointestinal-diseases).

Chapter 3
Distinguishing Benign Symptoms from Red Flags

What Makes a Symptom "Benign"?

The Different Meanings of "Benign": Context Matters

In the field of healthcare, the word "benign" generally has two meanings, depending on the context.

Context 1: distinguishing between either benign or sinister. In this context, something benign is something that is not harmful and thus not a threat to one's life in the short- or long-term. Along the same lines, it's also something that typically does not progress or worsen, at least not to a clinically significant degree. An example would be a skin tag on a person's back; these small fleshy protuberances don't bleed, cause pain, or grow in size.

Context 2: distinguishing between either benign or malignant, i.e. cancerous. In this context, something benign is something that is not cancerous. An example would be a hemorrhoid; hemorrhoids are veins around the anus that may become enlarged but do not have the potential to turn into cancer.

Potential Confusion Surrounding the Term "Benign"

There admittedly is room for confusion to arise with the term "benign" given it has two potential meanings. Additionally, there are two facets that may cause additional confusion:

1. Benign doesn't always mean not causing symptoms. Indeed, some problems that are benign can be quite unpleasant, painful, or otherwise bothersome. For example, an external hemorrhoid can become clotted and cause exquisite pain.

J. H. Tabibian, *Digestive Problems Solved*,
https://doi.org/10.1007/978-3-031-16317-3_3

However, it's still benign in the sense that it's not cancerous (context 2) and it almost never is a threat to one's life (context 1).

2. Benign is sometimes used to characterize conditions that are not yet cancer but can eventually become cancer. An example is an adenoma, a type of colon polyp, or wart-like fleshy growth. Adenomas, or adenomatous polyps, are a common finding in the colon and are technically "dysplastic" by definition. That is, they embody a middle ground between being benign and being cancerous. If left unremoved and allowed to grow for years, they can progress to become colon cancer. So on the one hand they are benign given they are not yet malignant, but it should be recognized that that an adenomatous polyp in the colon is a precancerous polyp. Context 2 is therefore sometimes split into three categories to be more technically correct: benign, dysplastic or "pre-malignant", and malignant.

What Are "Red Flags" in Medicine?

Red flags are findings that, as one might expect, set off an alert or alarm in a health-care provider's mind. They indicate potential for a sinister and possibly malignant underlying process and thus merit expedited and sometimes urgent evaluation. This can apply to all sorts of problems, digestive and otherwise. What specifically constitutes a red flag finding may depend on the context; for instance, red flags in someone with a headache will be somewhat different than red flags in someone with rectal area pain, and this is because the two are anatomically and functionally distinct. Red flags in someone with a headache may include visual changes and speech deficits, potentially representing an underlying brain cancer or severe inflammation of the brain, whereas red flags in someone with rectal area pain may be blood in the stool and weight loss, potentially representing an underlying colon cancer.

Within the realm of digestive problems, there are several red flags to bear in mind, as shown in Table 3.1. Even within the focused context of digestive problems,

Table 3.1 Red flags in the context of digestive problems

Finding
Unintentional weight loss
New-onset symptoms above age 45–50 years
Vomiting
Blood in stool/in toilet bowl or black stools
Pain or other symptom waking up from sleep
Early satiety (feeling full quickly)
Fever

Note: Other findings not included here may represent red flags in some scenarios, and not all of these findings always equate to a sinister underlying problem.

though, red flags can vary quite a bit given how vast the digestive system is. For example, red flags to look out for in someone with difficulty swallowing would include vomiting, blood in the vomit, and unintentional weight loss, whereas in someone with constipation, red flags would include blood in the stool, unintentional weight loss, and anemia. This example illustrates that while there can be variation in what constitutes a red flag in a given case, there can also be some overlap.

"Red Flags" don't Always Indicate Doom and Gloom

It's important to recognize that many times individuals with a red flag or multiple red flags don't have a sinister or malignant underlying disease, as illustrated in Fig. 3.1. However, because suspicion is raised when a red flag is present, it's

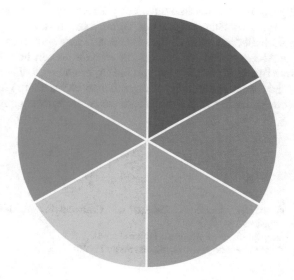

- Benign findings and benign problem
- Benign findings and sinister problem
- Red flag findings and benign problem
- Red flag findings and sinister problem
- No symptoms and benign problem
- No symptoms and sinister problem

Fig. 3.1 Different combinations of symptoms and underlying problems among patients with a digestive problem.
Legend: Pie slices can vary in size depending on the patient population and the particular digestive problem. Overall this figure points to the discordance there can be between the nature of a patient's findings or symptoms and the nature of the underlying problem

important to take timely steps to further investigate. After all, you generally don't know until you take a look into and investigate the matter.

On the flip side, the absence of red flags doesn't always mean that a sinister or malignant process is not present. Indeed, this is one of the major challenges in making an early diagnosis of a variety of different diseases, including cancers. For example, individuals with early stage colon cancer often have no symptoms—no visible blood in the stool, no weight loss, and no anemia. This is precisely the reason why screening programs have been created. Colon cancer is a hallmark disease wherein screening can result in earlier diagnosis, if not outright prevention, and save lives.

Putting it all Together

If you have digestive problems that have not yet been evaluated, it is advisable to seek evaluation from a healthcare provider. Going a step further, if you have any red flags, you should seek evaluation all the sooner and make sure to convey these findings to your provider so that the appropriate evaluation can be undertaken in an appropriate time frame. Knowing why you are experiencing a digestive problem is empowering. The causes and triggers of digestive problems are the focus of the next section of the book, starting with genes, food, the environment and more as covered in Chap. 4.

Further Reading

Common GI symptoms. American College of Gastroenterology. https://gi.org/topics/common-gi-symptoms/.
When to call a doctor for digestive problems (webmd.com).
When to call the doctor about digestive problems. Sutter Health.

Part II
Triggers and Causes of Digestive Problems: A Broad Spectrum of Possibilities

Chapter 4
Genes, Food, Environment, and Beyond

Digestive problems can be caused or worsened by a long list of things, depending on the individual and the specific problem in question. Let's collectively refer to these things as "triggers". Sometimes there is one clear trigger, other times there are multiple triggers, and other times the trigger is unclear. To provide a conceptual framework, it can be helpful to organize triggers into categories; one way to do so is to categorize them as being intrinsic, extrinsic, or behavioral. In this chapter, I aim to provide an overview of these categories and explore several of the triggers within each of them, including but not limited to the role of our genetic makeup, the foods we eat, our environment, our behaviors, and more. An understanding of these and other potential triggers is important for comprehension of one's digestive problem as well as identifying appropriate treatment options.

What Types of Things can Trigger Digestive Problems?

So many different things can trigger digestive problems—the sky is essentially the limit. What's more, even a single digestive problem can have different triggers in different individuals. Though as patients and providers we generally want to know what the trigger of digestive problem is, it can be quite difficult in some cases. In fact, and as I'll discuss later in this chapter, many times the trigger may not be identified, even after extensive testing. As presented in Table 4.1, I often find it useful to conceptualize triggers of digestive problems into three broad categories:

- Intrinsic: based on your genes, your DNA, or something else inside and innate to your body
- Extrinsic: based on the things around you, from the food you eat to the medications you take and so forth, or
- Behavioral: based on your lifestyle habits

J. H. Tabibian, *Digestive Problems Solved*, https://doi.org/10.1007/978-3-031-16317-3_4

Table 4.1 Triggers of digestive problems in a summarized framework of intrinsic, extrinsic, and behavioral factors

Intrinsic
Genetics
Aging
Pregnancy
Menstrual cycle
Obesity
Microbiome
Extrinsic
Food
Water
Air
Chemicals
Medications
Behavioral
Psychosocial issues
Mental illness
Cultural considerations
Lifestyle habits

Legend: The term "trigger" is used loosely here and can refer to underlying causes as well as aggravating or worsening factors. This list is not exhaustive; in addition, some factors may span across more than one category (e.g. obesity may be intrinsic, extrinsic, and/or behavioral)

As we are living, breathing, moving organisms, there's no question that these triggers interact with and influence (to amplify or suppress) each other. As a result, while you are reading this chapter, you may stop and think, "wait a minute, is that really intrinsic?" or "how is that really extrinsic?", and it's quite possible you have a valid point. The bounds between these categories can be blurry, and there can be overlap. For instance, obesity is a trigger for many digestive problems, acid gastroesophageal reflux and gallstones being common examples. Obesity has been considered an intrinsic condition, but is it really? Is it not due to both intrinsic and non-intrinsic factors? I would say it is often hard to say definitively and can vary from individual to individual.

Ultimately, how intrinsic, extrinsic, and behavioral triggers come together in a given individual is what ultimately determines whether or not a problem, digestive or otherwise, will actually arise, how severe it may be, and so forth. Let's explore each of these three categories. As a forewarning, this is a foundational and thus long chapter.

Intrinsic Factors

For many digestive problems, it is necessary to have some sort of underlying intrinsic predisposition. Intrinsic refers to something that originates or is present from within, whether it is genetically-based or otherwise. Some intrinsic factors are present and lead to problems from birth, whereas others have an onset later on in life. The examples are innumerable, thus I will discuss a few main broad subcategories and a few specific examples.

Genetics

Many digestive problems are genetically-based in one way or another. Sometimes it is just a genetic predisposition to having a certain problem, meaning you may or may not develop it depending on other factors. On the other hand, a person can have a specific genetic mutation or change that directly causes a problem, such as an inherited colon cancer syndrome, hereditary hemochromatosis. Overall, this latter scenario (i.e. having a specific genetic mutation or change) is responsible for only a minority of cases of digestive problems. Still, as they constitute an important subset, it is essential for the evaluating healthcare provider to keep these in mind and rule them out as deemed clinically appropriate. The more common scenario, the genetic predisposition, requires an additional trigger such as obesity, poor diet, or smoking for a digestive problem to actually develop. For example, a person may have a genetic predisposition for forming gallstones, which when coupled with a diet high in unhealthy fat and cholesterol, leads to the development of gallstones. Unfortunately, we can't really change our genetic predisposition, but many times we can change or otherwise mitigate the additional triggers.

While in the subcategory of genetic factors, I should make mention of a newer field of research, which is called epigenetics. The epigenome refers to modifications that are made to our genes, including the addition of extra molecules that can have different signaling functions, rather than just the genes themselves. These modifications can be the triggers of various digestive problems (or so it seems, but much more research is needed). While not genetic or hereditary in the traditional sense, epigenetics can be considered an intrinsic process, albeit modifiable by extrinsic factors, such as what we eat or exposure to pollutants.

Aging

Myriad changes occur in the human body with age, and the GI system is not exempt from these. Just like your skin can become thinner, more delicate, and wrinkled over time, similar anatomical and structural changes can occur in the GI system. In addition, the way our GI system functions can change with age. For example, our intestinal "thermostat" may change such that things run slower, potentially resulting in constipation; we may not digest certain substances, like lactose, as well as before, resulting in gas, bloating, and/or diarrhea; sphincter muscles may become weaker, resulting in acid reflux or, at the other end, fecal incontinence; and so forth. Our lifestyles also change with age, so we may not be eating the same or being as active as we once had, which compounds matters. One of the tricky aspects of age-related change is that some is expected and part of the "normal" aging process, whereas some is due to something more sinister, such as development of a disease, sometimes even cancer. For this reason, many clinical guidelines factor in age, such that a given symptom plus age above a certain cutoff, such as 45 or 60 years, merits more thorough and expeditious evaluation than if the symptom was to occur in a younger individual (in whom cancer would be statistically much less likely). This is to say, age above a certain threshold may be considered a red flag in the setting of a new-onset problem.

Pregnancy

Anyone who has been pregnant or knows about symptoms which can arise during pregnancy can attest to the various changes that happen to the body, some of them being the onset or worsening of digestive problems. This is multi-factorial but in large part driven by alterations in several hormones, including but not limited to progesterone. Progesterone is known for causing constipation during pregnancy by slowing the motility, or the rhythmic contraction of muscles, of the GI tract. The digestive system is quite sensitive to hormonal changes; during pregnancy, it's common for digestive problems such as nausea, reflux, and constipation to worsen, but in other (less common) cases there can be improvements. While these problems can be very bothersome, they are often expected, treatable, and resolve post-partum.

Menstrual Cycle

Periods can bring on a slew of unpleasant symptoms, and these can be mental, emotional, physical, and yes, also pertaining to the GI system. Indeed, many if not most women experience more digestive problems like gas, bloating, diarrhea, and/or constipation during their period. Analogous to pregnancy, these are largely due to fluctuations in levels of hormones and other signaling molecules, such as prostaglandins. In fact, the same signaling molecules that trigger periods also have effects on the GI system, as different cell types in the GI system have receptors for estrogen, progesterone, and prostaglandins. In contrast to progesterone, estrogen tends to enhance GI motility and can be to blame for more frequent stools or even diarrhea when levels increase. And as many would affirm, there can be changes during other times in the cycle, not just during or right before menses. Overall, the points I want to make here are that as with pregnancy, digestive problems during the menstrual cycle may be expected (albeit bothersome) and in a sense are perhaps not really digestive problems but rather gynecological hormonal changes manifesting in the GI system. Thus, it's important to pay attention to what the symptoms are, when they are occurring during the cycle, and sharing this information with your primary care provider, gynecologist, and/or gastroenterologist to try to come up with a treatment plan. Some women may benefit from hormonal contraception, like birth control pills or a hormonal IUD, to help regulate the hormonal fluctuations that trigger digestive problems associated with the menstrual cycle, though many other treatments, including herbal remedies, over-the-counter medications, and mind-body interventions, exist and may be considered.

Extrinsic Factors

Essentially everything around us and/or that we are exposed to constitutes an extrinsic factor. Thus, it should be no surprise that the list of triggers in this category is long: food, water, air, sun, chemicals (including cigarettes, alcohol, environmental pollutants), medications, the intestinal microbiome (discussed in Chap. 6), and more. Any and all of these, directly or indirectly, can have an influence on digestive health and whether or not problems arise. How much influence they might have depends on the individual, but I will say that overall, based on my experience as a physician and a patient, the influence can be major in a considerable proportion of cases. A few examples of how some extrinsic factors may play into and serve as triggers of digestive problems are discussed below.

Food

With regard to food, it has been said that "you are what you eat." I would change this slightly to say "what you eat can determine your health and how you feel." To use the analogy of a car, you pump gas into it, and the gas affects how the car runs. If you use the wrong octane, there can be combustion issues, as a result of which the car may not run well or may even be unsafe. The same goes with the food we put into our system. Food may be perhaps the most common trigger of digestive problems, yet many individuals tend to overlook its importance. For example, one morning when I woke up I felt a sensation of heartburn, or burning just under my sternum, and I thought to myself, "Oh, why am I experiencing this? What's going on? This may not be good." It wasn't until a couple hours later that I remembered I had eaten a large amount of pepperoni pizza with pickled jalapeño peppers the night before. Between the red sauce, which is acidic, the fat from the cheese and pepperoni, which causes the stomach to empty at a slower rate, and the spice in the pepperoni and jalapeños, it should be no surprise that I experienced heartburn. Yet, I had completely forgotten about the pizza, and here I am a gastroenterologist. Suffice it to say, it's very easy to lose track of the things we eat that can account for the problems we experience. In the medical setting, associations between digestive problems and food are one of the first things we ask about and explore when trying to make a diagnosis so it's very much worth giving it adequate thought. Food triggers (intolerances and others) are more common than people think, and identifying them is crucial to managing digestive problems, as discussed further in Chap. 12.

Water

Water is essential to life and in fact is the major constituent of our bodies, making up nearly 60%. Insufficient intake of water can lead to much more than just dry mouth or a sense of thirst; it can trigger heartburn, constipation, kidney injury, and other negative downstream effects. Water is a carrier for substances that we may not want to be ingesting (e.g. contaminants); thus, where clean drinking water is scarce, digestive and other problems abound. Unfortunately, we often times don't know what unwanted substances may be in our drinking water On the bright side, our body has mechanisms to effectively cope with many of these. All in all, while I don't advise patients to only drink Evian water, I do think that we sometimes take the cleanliness of water for granted. On that note, if you travel and develop a digestive problem while drinking local water, consider the water source, and infectious organisms such as the parasite *Giardia* that may be in it, as a potential trigger.

Air

The air we breathe may seem to be related to the respiratory tract rather than the digestive tract, but in fact it is related to both. Some of what we breathe is swallowed, enters the esophagus, and goes on down through the digestive tract. Moreover, what we breathe can be absorbed into the bloodstream and circulated throughout the body, including to the gastrointestinal system. For these reasons, it makes sense that some respiratory illnesses that are associated with digestive problems; for example, asthma is associated with a condition known as "eosinophilic esophagitis."

Chemicals

Chemicals are a vast topic. In the interest of brevity and practicality, I will focus on tobacco and alcohol, though food additives and contaminants are also a noteworthy subject. Both tobacco and alcohol have numerous, well-described associations with a greater risk of health problems, digestive and otherwise. The list is long and can include anything from pancreas cancer to stomach ulcers to worsening of various existing conditions. Still, it oftentimes doesn't occur to individuals that the digestive problems they are experiencing can be triggered by tobacco or alcohol. Identifying a chemical as a trigger of a digestive problem offers an opportunity for intervention, difficult as it may be. If you smoke or drink, even if not in excess, it's worth asking your provider if it could be acting as a trigger in your case.

Medications

This is a broad and important category that can be easily overlooked by patients as well as providers, for a number of reasons. It includes prescription and over-the-counter medications as well as complementary and alternative medicines (CAMs). Generally speaking, for prescription and over-the-counter medications, adverse side effect profiles and statistics are well known, though it is often unknown which patients will or will not experience them and when, so vigilance is essential. It should be said here that some of the best-studied and important medications, while generally safe, can have GI and other adverse side effects in a small but not insignificant proportion of patients. Moreover, even medications intended to treat digestive problems can trigger *other* digestive problems. For instance, some acid suppression medicines can trigger diarrhea, which in people who have constipation may be a great side effect, but in those who have normal bowel habits, can be untoward. This underscores the importance of being vigilant for medication-induced adverse side effects.

To quickly touch upon CAMs, though many have been around for centuries or more, they generally have not been as rigorously tested, and thus their adverse side effect profile is typically less known. Compounding this issue are the different carriers and preservatives that may be combined with the active ingredient of a CAM. In other words, just because something is a CAM doesn't always mean it's safe, at least not in every person. In addition, drug-drug interactions can occur with Western medicine, and different people have different sensitivities or predispositions to these. I would be lying if I said I have not seen serious and even life-threatening complications from seemingly safe CAMs. CAMs are discussed further as the focus of Chap. 14.

Behavioral Factors

This category is interesting in part because it is perhaps the most susceptible to being considered taboo or irrelevant in the context of digestive problems. Though there are many ways to conceptualize or subcategorize behavioral factors, I think a pragmatic approach would be to think of them along the following lines: i) mental health and psychosocial issues, ii) cultural considerations, and iii) lifestyle habits. Entire books can be written on just one of these three subcategories, and as all three are under the behavioral factors umbrella, they tend to have substantial interdependence and overlap. In the interest of pragmatism and focus, I will share just a few high-level tidbits.

All three of these subcategories are salient for two main reasons: they can influence how and when a digestive problem develops, and they may make an existing digestive problem better or worse. What's more, they can also impact treatment decisions in terms of determining which treatment is best suited for a given patient. I'd like to herein provide a few examples I have come across in my professional experience that touch upon these three behavioral subcategories.

Mental Health and Psychosocial Issues

Mental health issues, such as depression, can trigger digestive problems in addition to making them more difficult to cope with. When coping mechanisms fall short, symptoms become amplified, making problems more bothersome and seemingly worse than they objectively may be. Moreover, there is a bi-directional relationship; that is, digestive problems can also make mental health issues worse. Just imagine how a person suffering from depression would feel if the discomfort of constipation or acid reflux were added on to his or her plate.

Like mental health issues, psychosocial variables such as turbulence at home and perceived stress can similarly have a negative impact on digestive problems, and vice-versa. Trying to address digestive problems without keeping mental health and psychosocial factors in sight (and adequately managed) creates vulnerable gaps in care and impediments to wellness for patients and providers, as discussed further in Chap. 7.

Cultural Considerations

If nothing else, cultural variables can influence how a digestive problem is perceived and managed. The stronger your cultural ties, the stronger this influence may be. For instance, I recall having seen patients who, seemingly for cultural reasons, manifested their life stress in their chest by feeling short of breath or in their abdomen by feeling nausea or discomfort. Conversely, I've also had patients who attributed their abdominal pain and weight loss to benign or coincidental processes and who were unwilling to see the objective evidence of a more sinister condition nor to allow medical care. Cultural variables may also determine the perceived appropriateness of and amenability to a recommended treatment. Suffice it to say, cultural variables can be quite fascinating and relevant in this regard.

Lifestyle Habits

Lifestyle habits include things such as sleep, bowel, and eating patterns and tendencies. For many individuals, lifestyle habits are an important consideration with regard to understanding and managing digestive problems. As fundamental aspects of how we live, they can play a role in almost any digestive problem and are also interrelated with each other. Take sleep for instance: too much or too little sleep, or otherwise abnormal sleep patterns such as difficulty falling asleep or frequent awakenings, can impact what time you eat, what is available to eat, your appetite, and your bowel movement schedule. As another example, if you don't move your bowels regularly and appropriately, perhaps because you don't make time for it in your day or don't have the urge, you may feel bloated, anxious about when your bowel movement may come next, or not hungry due to a sense of fullness, just to name a few potential consequences. And as a third example of lifestyle habits, imagine how your eating tendencies may impact your digestive and overall wellness; for instance, eating too late can predispose to acid reflux, eating too fast can lead to overeating, belching, queasiness, or other adverse outcomes, and eating too infrequently can lead to hunger pains, unintentional weight loss, or binge eating. Overall, the effects of lifestyle habits are far-reaching.

Caveats Regarding the Relationship Between Triggers and Digestive Problems

There are two important points I would like to mention that are salient when we think about potential triggers:

- Sometimes a trigger—be it intrinsic, extrinsic, or behavioral– is present but isn't really the cause of or otherwise related to the problem; it's just coincidental
- Sometimes a trigger is present, but we don't have the tools, i.e. the diagnostic tests or technology, to detect or prove it

With regard to the first point, an example would be having Type 2 diabetes and nausea. Some patients with diabetes can experience digestive problems such as nausea. In some of these patients, the diabetes is in fact the trigger, especially if it's not well-controlled. For example, the patient may have diabetic gastroparesis from years of high blood sugar levels. But in many patients, the diabetes is not the trigger, it's simply coincidental with the digestive problem. To put this into perspective with another example, imagine you have a hiatal hernia, where the stomach slips up above the diaphragm (Fig. 4.1). This condition is very common—nearly 1 in 5 adults have a hiatal hernia—and can predispose to gastroesophageal reflux disease (GERD) given it makes it easier for gastric contents to go back up into the esophagus. However, not everyone who has a hiatal hernia suffers from GERD, nor does everyone with GERD have a hiatal hernia.

With regard to the second point, many times there is a trigger present, but we as a medical community don't have the tools, tests, or technology to detect or prove it. When a problem is present but doesn't seem to have an explanation, we may refer to it in medical lexicon as "idiopathic." To provide an example, some patients with constipation may have abnormal function of their intestinal pacemaker cells, known as the "interstitial cells of Cajal." Whether it's genetic or due to some other trigger, the cells work more slowly in such patients and thus bowel movements happen less

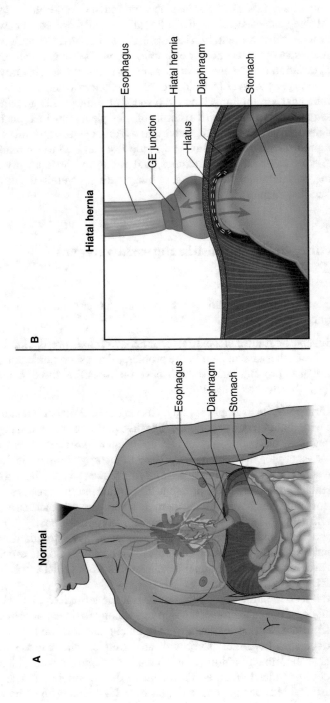

Fig. 4.1 Hiatal hernia: a risk factor for gastroesophageal reflux.
Legend: A. Normal anatomy showing the esophagus joining the stomach at the esophagogastric junction, which is located at the level of the diaphragm; note how the stomach is located completely below the diaphragm. B. A zoomed in view showing a sliding hiatal hernia, wherein the top (i.e. proximal) portion of the stomach slides above the hiatus, or opening, of the diaphragm. A hiatal hernia compromises the overall integrity of the esophagogastric junction, as discussed in Chap. 1, and can thus predispose to reflux of gastric contents up into the esophagus

frequently. However, we currently don't have the tools to make this determination or diagnosis, therefore, we may simply refer to the constipation as "idiopathic". This lack of tools actually applies to a broader array of problems than what one may recognize which is potentially problematic in that a targeted treatment to address the underlying cause can't be administered, and thus treatment becomes "symptomatic" or "empiric". That is, we're left with trying our best to remedy a problem based on what its symptoms are and what we think the underlying cause may possibly be. Though this might not be ideal, if done thoughtfully, it can be quite effective. For instance, we can't always determine why someone's stomach is producing excess acid, but we have medications which can decrease acid production and thus effectively manage problems that it may be causing.

Putting it all Together

Triggers of digestive problems, whether they are the initial cause of or something that worsens a given problem, can be conceptualized as being intrinsic, extrinsic, or behavioral. In any individual patient, and for essentially any problem, there may be just one trigger or (more often) a combination of triggers. Triggers are quite varied: some are more "potent" than others, some are more reversible than others, some are easier to identify than others, and so forth. In this chapter we discussed some of the main factors in each of the three trigger categories, but the possibilities are endless. When you develop a digestive problem, it is of critical importance to think about what the potential triggers may be. Not infrequently, you'll be able to come up with some triggers on your own, and using the framework of intrinsic, extrinsic, or behavioral can be a useful tool for this. You might realize, for instance, that your heartburn is linked directly to your eating habits and that you only feel it when you eat a late meal or drink red wine. Generally speaking, though, it's prudent to work with your healthcare provider to most accurately identify and manage triggers that you may not be aware of. Your healthcare provider can help you clarify, for example, what really is a trigger versus what is just a coincidence with regard to your digestive problem and accordingly develop a care plan. Having this expanded perspective and understanding about your digestive problem will provide substantive value in gaining direction, peace of mind, and determining the most fitting management options.

As we continue along within this section of the book, we will build upon the framework provided herein and explore some additional topics with regard to triggers of digestive problems. With this in mind, being as the digestive tract is a long, tubular structure with an entrance and exit point, issues with flow can sometimes arise, and these in turn can constitute the trigger of a digestive problem. These flow issues are covered next in Chap. 5.

Further Reading

Aerophagia in adults: a comparison with functional dyspepsia. PubMed (nih.gov).
Crosstalk between the microbiome and epigenome: messages from bugs (nih.gov).
Epigenetic mechanisms in irritable bowel syndrome (nih.gov).
Gastrointestinal symptoms before and during menses in healthy women. PubMed (nih.gov).
Genetics in gastroenterology: what you need to know, part 1. Consultant360.
https://familydoctor.org/condition/indigestion-dyspepsia/
https://gastro.org/guidelines/
https://gi.org/guidelines/
https://gi.org/topics/common-gi-problems-in-women/
https://medlineplus.gov/genetics/understanding/howgeneswork/epigenome/#:~:text=
    Environmental%20influences%2C%20such%20as%20a%20person%E2%80%99s%20
    diet%20and,cells%2C%20ensuring%20that%20only%20necessary%20proteins%20are%20
    produced
Irritable bowel syndrome and functional dyspepsia: different diseases or a single disorder with
    different manifestations? PubMed (nih.gov).
Multicultural aspects in functional gastrointestinal disorders (FGIDs). Gastroenterology (gastro-
    journal.org).
The effect of cigarette smoking on salivation and esophageal acid clearance. PubMed (nih.gov).

Chapter 5
Flow Problems: Digestive Tract Blockages and Dysmotility

The digestive tract is at the center of the GI system and is essentially a long and complex tubular passageway, as discussed in Chap. 1. Many digestive problems are attributable to issues in how things flow through this passageway. As you may imagine, an issue with flow in one place can generate upstream or downstream issues, so it's important to think about the system as a whole. In this chapter I aim to present an overview of digestive tract flow and discuss how issues with digestive tract flow can serve as potential triggers of digestive problems.

What Causes Problems with GI Flow

For the digestive tract to function normally, things need to go through, be processed, and come out the other end properly. This "flow", if you will, can go wrong when there is one or both of the following issues at play: (1) a blockage or (2) abnormal function, called dysmotility. Think of the digestive tract as an automotive assembly line: its flow can become disrupted if (1) a huge mechanical hindrance such as a boulder is placed somewhere along the way (blockage) or (2) if the person in charge of transferring the wheels to the car decides to stop doing their job (dysmotility). Blockages can be of varying degrees and types; patients who develop a complete blockage are usually hospitalized and may require an emergency surgery or procedure to relieve the blockage. Motility problems are usually chronic/longstanding and don't typically require emergenty care, though they may in rare cases.

As with an assembly line, there are many specific reasons why and places where our digestive tract can have flow problems.

© The Author(s), under exclusive license to Springer Nature Switzerland AG 2023
J. H. Tabibian, *Digestive Problems Solved*,
https://doi.org/10.1007/978-3-031-16317-3_5

Digestive Tract Blockage

The technical term for a blockage is an "obstruction". A blockage of the digestive tract can occur just about anywhere, from esophagus to rectum. Certain causes of blockage are more common in certain areas, so there is variation in what the cause may be according to the anatomical location within the digestive tract. Blockages can be classified in several different ways, and there is some overlap between them. The classifications can also be (and are often) used in conjunction.

- **Benign vs. malignant obstruction**: In this classification, an obstruction is either due to a benign, noncancerous condition or a malignant, cancerous condition. In the colon, for instance, most obstructions are malignant, such as due to colorectal cancer. Indeed, roughly a quarter of patients with colorectal cancer have obstruction as their presenting symptom. Benign causes are many and depend in part on where in the digestive tract the obstruction is. To list a few examples, benign causes of obstruction include volvulus, intussusception, hernia, scarring, Crohn's disease, and diverticulitis. Several of these present suddenly and constitute an emergency, whereas others may be more insidious. Generally, X-rays or more sophisticated imaging studies such as computed tomography (CT) will be needed to help determine if an obstruction is benign or malignant and to determine the specific underlying cause.
- **Acute vs. chronic**: In this classification, an obstruction is characterized based on how long it has been apparent. Some obstructions are acute and occur relatively suddenly; these typically require urgent or emergent intervention, e.g. surgery. In other cases, such as when there is cancer that has spread to the abdomen, obstruction can be a chronic issue. Some acute causes of obstruction can become recurrent, each time lasting for a relatively short period of time.
- **Intrinsic vs. extrinsic**: In this classification, an obstruction is characterized as either arising from within the digestive tract (i.e. intrinsic) or from something outside the digestive tract (i.e. extrinsic). A mass that is growing inside the stomach that eventually blocks off the flow of food and liquid through the pylorus would be an example of an intrinsic obstruction. On the other hand, scar tissue on the outside of the small bowel known as adhesions or a uterine tumor pressing on the small bowel would be examples of an extrinsic obstruction. In most cases, if the cause of an obstruction is extrinsic to the digestive tract, it will not be a gastroenterologist who treats it (may instead require a surgeon).
- **Partial vs. complete**: In this classification, an obstruction is characterized as either being a partial or a complete blockage, depending on the severity of obstruction. In the former, some things can still get through, just not to a normal degree. In the latter, the blockage is so severe that essentially nothing can get through; even water can't get through the esophagus, if a complete esophageal

obstruction, and even gas cannot get through the rectum, if a complete rectal obstruction. Depending on the underlying cause, some partial obstructions can become complete over time. For example, if a mass is causing a partial obstruction and something, such as chemotherapy, radiation, surgery, or a stent, isn't done to address the mass, the obstruction can eventually become complete.

- **Location (esophagus vs. stomach vs. small bowel vs. colon):** In this classification, the emphasis is placed on where the obstruction is located, putting aside whether or not it's malignant, acute, intrinsic, partial, or other. In a sense, this is the most practical way to begin when classifying an obstruction, since it's often the first thing that will be known to the healthcare provider after initial evaluation and imaging. For example, an X-ray or CT scan may show a small bowel obstruction, but it's only with further investigation and data acquisition that one can determine if it is benign or not, intrinsic or not, and so forth. Another benefit of this classification is that it narrows down the differential diagnosis, as certain causes of obstruction can only occur in certain organs. For instance, a lung mass is probably not going to be the cause of a small bowel obstruction, but it could indeed cause esophageal obstruction. Conversely, an inguinal or abdominal wall hernia is not going to be the cause of esophageal obstruction, but it could certainly cause small or large bowel obstruction.

Digestive Tract Dysmotility

In practical terms, dysmotility refers to a problem with function rather than form or structure (see Chap. 1 for more information regarding functional disorders). Picture a Ferrari that you are looking at from across the street. The car looks terrific and has genuine form and structure, but if the chip inside that controls the engine isn't working, the car isn't going to move as you would expect. Normal digestive tract motility is a complex phenomenon that requires coordination of the sympathetic, parasympathetic, and enteric nervous systems, specialized pacemaker cells called the "interstitial cells of Cajal", and smooth muscle cells of the digestive tract. If any one of these goes awry in any location, a dysmotility may occur. Dysmotility can mean that contractions or some other function are occurring too infrequently, too frequently, too weakly, too strongly, or in some other abnormal manner. The symptoms of dysmotility by and large mimic those of obstruction. Thus if a patient presents with what seems to be a flow problem, such as vomiting up food or only defecating once a week, it's nearly impossible to know, without further testing, if there is a blockage or a dysmotility. Additionally, because of the functional nature of dysmotility, it can sometimes be more difficult to treat; for example, there isn't a mass to cut out or a hernia to repair.

What Are the Symptoms of Flow Problems?

The symptoms caused by a flow problem depend on the nature of the flow problem, in particular where it is, how severe it is, and what the underlying cause is (Fig. 5.1). If the problem is in the esophagus, the most common symptoms or manifestations are difficulty swallowing, feeling like food is getting stuck, and/or chest pain with eating. Of course, chest pain can be due to heart, lung, or other problems, so context is important. If a flow problem in the esophagus is severe, vomiting or regurgitation may be a symptom, and eventually even weight loss due to not enough calories being taken in. At the other end of the digestive tract, in the colon, a flow problem

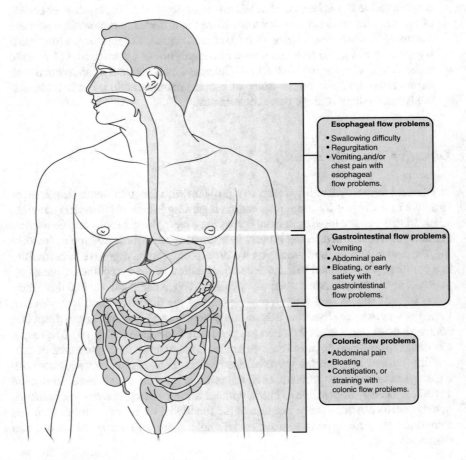

Fig. 5.1 Digestive tract flow problems and associated symptoms

may manifest as constipation, difficulty evacuating one's bowels (e.g. having to strain), and/or bloating. There may also be abdominal pain, nausea, and even vomiting (which people don't always associate with the lower part of the digestive tract). Indeed, many individuals have bloating and nausea, but once modifications are made to help them to evacuate their bowels regularly and effectively address the flow problem in the digestive tract (especially the colon), their symptoms go away. This exemplifies the importance of considering the digestive tract as a whole continuous system. On a related note, though beyond the scope of discussion here, flow problems can also exist in the accessory organs, in particular the gallbladder (including the bile ducts leading to and away from it) and the pancreatic ducts; when present, they can cause symptoms that may mimic flow problems in the digestive tract, especially in the stomach and small intestine. Conversely, symptoms due to flow (or other) problems in the stomach and small intestine can mimic problems of the gallbladder and pancreas.

Bloating: A Common Problem that Is Sometimes but Not Always Due to Flow Issues

Bloating is a very common digestive problem that may be due to the flow issues I've mentioned thus far. Importantly, bloating can mean different things to different individuals, and not all bloating is the same. Because of how ubiquitous a problem it is, it deserves special mention. Some people refer to excess belching, or excess flatulence, or a protuberant abdomen as bloating; these are all quite different issues. This impacts what the potential causes and treatments of a case of "bloating" may be. Thus, in general, I like to take a step back and conceptualize bloating as a fundamental problem with any of the following three factors:

- excessive air swallowing, or aerophagia,
- increased intraluminal production of gas, or too much gas being produced within the intestines, or
- abnormal dissipation of gas, or inappropriate absorption or expulsion of gas.

Aerophagia

It is normal to swallow or ingest a small amount of air (primarily nitrogen and oxygen). This happens, for instance, with swallowing and with laughing. The amount of air swallowed in these scenarios is fairly negligible, on the order of a few milliliters. Larger amounts of air may be swallowed in certain scenarios. These include gulping food, drinking from a bottle or straw, smoking, and stress/anxiety. Thus, when bloating is a problem, attention needs to be turned to the potential role of aerophagia in causing or worsening the process.

Increased Production of Gas

In addition to nitrogen and oxygen which are swallowed, there are three principal gases that are produced within the intestines: carbon dioxide, hydrogen, and methane. These gases are produced by intestinal bacteria as a byproduct of their metabolic activity during the digestion of the fats, proteins, and carbohydrates that we ingest. In the case of methane, it is predominantly produced by the bacterium *Methanobrevibacter smithii*, which carries out the reaction: $4H_2 + CO_2 -- > CH_4 + 2H_2 0$. This reaction reduces the volume of gas particles that would otherwise be present in the colon. It should be noted that gas in the intestines is not a problem until it becomes a problem, which is often times a subjective call. If you begin to develop an excess of gas and bloating, it makes sense to first look at your diet as a potential cause. Some individuals will also try to manage their gas and bloating with probiotics, as will be discussed further in Chaps. 14 and 15, but this is a bit of a shot in the dark which may or may not lessen the production of gas in the intestines.

Abnormal Dissipation of Gas

This category primarily refers to problems with the flow of gas in the digestive tract, in particular due to either a blockage in the pipeline or a weakened barrier somewhere along it. Note that dysmotility can also be a contributing factor, though I wouldn't typically consider it a major factor per se. With regard to a blockage causing abnormal dissipation of gas, this can be the result of a few different things, including:

- Constipation, when copious amounts of solid stool pose an impediment to appropriate evacuation of gas;
- A mass, that is a benign or malignant tumor of some sort;
- A sharp angulation, as may be seen in patients with "adhesions", which are a form of scar tissue.

Though only the first of these is relatively common, all of these should be thought through in the patient with bloating not easily resolved with initial measures. With regard to a weakened barrier, the main one which can cause an issue with "bloating" is the gastroesophageal junction. When this natural barrier is weakened or laxed for whatever reason, air can travel upward and be expelled by excess belching rather than traveling down the digestive tract and being either absorbed into the bloodstream or expelled as normal flatus.

Putting it all Together

The digestive tract, the long and complex tubular passageway from mouth to rectum, is a foremost aspect of the gastrointestinal system (Chap. 1). There are many digestive problems that can be attributed to abnormal flow through this specialized passageway, which is generally due to either an obstruction (blockage) or a dysmotility (abnormal function). Obstruction and dysmotility, in turn, have many potential underlying causes, some better understood and more treatable than others. It should be noted that abnormal flow in one place, whatever the cause, can cause upstream or downstream problems, so it's necessary to think about the digestive tract from a global perspective. Bloating is one of many potential symptoms associated with abnormal flow, but it can also be due to other causes. Whether your digestive problem includes bloating or not, consideration of abnormal flow may be worthwhile as part of a comprehensive diagnostic approach.

So far in this book, we have covered a number of different triggers and causes of digestive problems. The role of the microbiome is covered next in Chap. 6.

Further Reading

Analysis of 230 cases of emergent surgery for obstructing colon cancer—lessons learned. PubMed (nih.gov).

Bowel obstruction and blockage: symptoms, causes, & treatment (webmd.com).

Clinical guideline: management of gastroparesis. PubMed (nih.gov).

Understanding an intestinal obstruction. Johns Hopkins Medicine.

Chapter 6
The Intestinal Microbiome: Friends, Foes, and Unknowns

A Primer on the Immune System: A Starting Point for Understanding the Microbiome

The immune system deals with various sources as well as types of microorganisms, including those on the surfaces we touch, the foods we eat, in the air we breathe, on our skin, and in our digestive tract. At a high level, the immune system is made up of two main parts that work together: the innate immune system, which provides a general, first-line defense, and the adaptive immune system, a more customized defense machinery. Though we will focus on the innate immune system going forward, it's worth mentioning that the adaptive immune system is not present at birth and that when it ultimately forms, it includes specialized immune cells and antibodies and handles things like remembering an old infection and being prepared to face it if encountered again.

As shown in Table 6.1, the innate immune system includes: (1) components of the host, including natural barriers such as our skin, mucous, and stomach acid, white blood cells such as macrophages and neutrophils, anti-microbial substances, and more, and (2) the compendium of resident microorganisms living on and in us. It may seem surprising that microorganisms comprise part of our innate immune system, but it's true. Not only that, but the good microorganisms fortunately make up the vast majority and are essential to our immune system, digestive wellness, and overall health.

What Constitutes the Intestinal Microbiome?

The intestinal microbiome refers to the collection of bacteria, fungi, and viruses and other micro-organisms that live in the digestive tract, particularly in the small and large intestine, as well as their metabolites and byproducts. The intestinal

© The Author(s), under exclusive license to Springer Nature Switzerland AG 2023
J. H. Tabibian, *Digestive Problems Solved*,
https://doi.org/10.1007/978-3-031-16317-3_6

Table 6.1 Overview of the main components of the human innate immune system

Host components
Physical barriers, such as skin, mucous, acidic gastric juices, tight junctions between cells
Antimicrobial proteins in and on the surface of certain cells
Inflammation-related proteins circulating in blood
Receptors on the surface of cells and circulating in blood that sense micro-organisms and signal a defense response
Cytokines and other mediators of the defense response released by immune cells
Immune cells such as macrophages, a type of white blood cell, that can engulf foreign material
The microbiome
Resident microorganisms: bacteria, fungi, viruses (and sometimes protozoans, parasites)
Metabolites of resident micro-organisms
Byproducts/particles of resident micro-organisms

microbiome's composition influences the maturation and effectiveness of the immune system, protects against bad microorganisms known as pathogens, and modulates inflammatory responses in order to maintain homeostasis, or balance. When the microbiome is in a healthy state, the term "eubiosis" is used to describe it. In contrast, "dysbiosis" refers to a change in the composition, diversity, and/or metabolites of the microbiome from a healthy state to one associated with disease or predisposing to disease.

When conceptualizing the microbiome, it's worth taking a moment to revisit something from earlier in this section of the book. In Chap. 4, we covered intrinsic, extrinsic, and behavioral factors as causes of digestive problems, we discussed how many of these factors can overlap or be interrelated; the microbiome is a prime example of this. On one hand, the microbiome is an intrinsic factor—after all, it is a part of our body. On the other hand, micro-organisms are not human cells, and new microorganisms can enter our body from the environment at any time. Further complicating this is the fact that the microbiome is an extremely dynamic entity. It is shaped by what we eat, what medications we take, what we do or don't do (like smoking and exercise), what health conditions we have, and so on, and can change over time-- even on a day-to-day basis to some degree. What's more, microbiome diversity varies in different parts of our bodies. The number and type of bacteria present in our small intestine is distinct compared to just a few inches downstream in the large intestine; when you have 25–30 feet of digestive tract, this essentially makes the microbiome possibilities all but endless. Going a step further, it's not only the abundance and composition of the microbiome that is relevant but also its function and how it impacts the function of the host, our body. The picture that I am hopefully painting here is the mind-boggling complexity and dynamic nature of the human microbiome.

What Is the Relationship Between the Intestinal Microbiome and Digestive Problems?

A disturbance to the healthy intestinal microbiome can lead to a broad array of digestive problems. The nature of such problems depends on the nature of the disturbance. To simplify, I generally categorize this relationship into one of three buckets:

- Infection with a specific pathogen that directly causes a digestive problem, such as:

  - *Salmonella*: a bacterium frequently associated with food poisoning, causes intestinal inflammation and a resultant diarrheal illness, usually resolving on its own
  - *C. difficile*: a bacterium often but not solely acquired in healthcare settings, causes colonic inflammation and resultant diarrheal illness, often prolonged and/or recurrent
  - *Norovirus*: a virus that is the most common cause of cruise ship-associated diarrheal outbreaks
  - *H. pylori*: a bacterium found in soil and other environmental sources that can live in and infect the stomach and cause inflammation and ulcers in the stomach or small intestine, among other issues, resulting in bloating and pain
  - *Candida*: a yeast, or type of fungus, which can cause white sores in the mouth known as thrush and/or can cause inflammation in the esophagus known as candida esophagitis
  - *Ascaris*: a parasitic worm whose eggs may be found in soil or on plants, and when ingested, leads to small intestinal infection, nutritional deficiency, and other health problems

- Dysbiosis that causes or contributes to a digestive problem, such as:

  - Small intestinal bacterial overgrowth (SIBO): a condition in which the small intestine is colonized by excessive amounts of aerobic and anaerobic bacteria. Irritable bowel syndrome, narcotic use, diabetes, and cirrhosis are associated with an increased risk of having SIBO.
  - Pouchitis: in patients who have had their entire colon removed, a pouch is often created using the small intestine to essentially recreate the rectum. Inflammation of this pouch is referred to as pouchitis, and it can be acute or chronic. Dysbiosis in the pouch and/or in the small intestine leading to the pouch is believed to be one of the key causes of pouchitis.

- Dysbiosis that is associated with a chronic digestive problem, such as:

  - Inflammatory bowel disease (IBD): IBD encompasses two main conditions, ulcerative colitis and Crohn's disease. IBD is a chronic inflammatory disorder of the intestinal tract, and patients with IBD have been found to have intestinal dysbiosis, with abnormally low levels of certain bacteria and abnormally high levels of others. The relationship is quite complex (far from being fully understood), but it seems there are changes that IBD causes in the microbiome, but there may also be some microbiome changes early on that lead to IBD. Of note, targeting the dysbiosis in IBD has been investigated as a treatment and continues to be an area of biomedical research.

– Primary sclerosing cholangitis (PSC): PSC is a chronic, inflammatory disorder of the bile ducts that results in their scarring and destruction. It has been termed the "black box" of liver disease since its cause remains enigmatic. Dysbiosis has been described in patients with PSC, but the nature and relevance of the relationship remain unclear. As with IBD, dysbiosis in PSC is an active area of research and may represent an area for therapeutic intervention; in fact, some studies have already reported significant benefits of treating PSC with specific antibiotics.

This three-bucket categorization condenses complex relationships between the microbiome and digestive problems into a simplified schema that applies to most patients whose digestive problems are related to a microbiome disturbance. But there are admittedly some patients and microbiome scenarios that may not neatly fit into a category. For instance, there are scenarios where a pathogen is present but does not cause a clinically apparent infection or other problem. As an example, there are thousands if not millions of people in the world with *H. pylori* present in their stomach, but not all of them have digestive problems; their body may have mechanisms to suppress the *H. pylori* and not let it cause inflammation, ulcers, abdominal pain, or other issues. But as long as the pathogen is present, it has the ability to cause problems when an imbalance arises that makes an individual more vulnerable. As another example, there are also individuals who are found to have dysbiosis and also have symptoms, but the symptoms are unrelated to the dysbiosis, despite the temptation to link the two.

What to Do about my Intestinal Microbiome

Despite what popular culture or the media may lead us to believe, microbiome research is still in its infancy. Thus, it is difficult to concretely say do this or that to make your microbiome healthy or to avoid dysbiosis. But there is some published research out there which indicates that certain foods and lifestyle habits are likely to promote a healthy microbiome. In random order, these include plants-based foods like fruits, vegetables, legumes, grains; foods rich in good microorganisms, or "probiotics," such as yogurt; and avoidance of foods high in animal fat, sugar, and additives. Until there is a more robust research base, specific recommendations are difficult if not impossible to confidently make. Within the confines of current scientific knowledge, Chap. 14 provides some pearls with regard to taking probiotics and modifying one's microbiome.

Putting it all Together

The intestinal microbiome refers to the collection of bacteria, fungi, and viruses as well as other microorganisms that live in our digestive tract, plus their metabolites and byproducts. The microbiome is part of our innate immune system and plays numerous vital roles in our overall health. Though our understanding of the microbiome is still very much evolving, it has been shown to play an essential role in the maturation and effectiveness of the immune system, protection against pathogens, and modulation of inflammatory responses—all with the central theme of maintaining host homeostasis. Though we do not have complete control over our microbiome, given some of it is determined by our genes, early life exposures, and so on, a healthy diet coupled with healthy living habits can help promote the formation and maintenance of a healthy microbiome. Disturbances to the microbiome may occur for a variety of reasons and can result in an unhealthy state, or dysbiosis, which represents one of many potential causes of digestive problems. Sometimes the relationship between dysbiosis and a digestive problem is clear cut—for example, an infection with *Salmonella* or *Norovirus* overwhelms the immune system and causes you to have diarrhea and nausea. Other times, however, it is difficult to understand. For instance, there are scenarios where there can be concomitant dysbiosis and digestive problems, and sometimes they are simply coincidental and unrelated to each other, so judicious interpretation is needed. Because dysbiosis is common and important in the context of digestive problems, it is important to consider it, test for it as clinically appropriate, and if present, manage it accordingly. This requires involvement of a healthcare provider, and often, a gastroenterologist.

So far in this section, we have covered many of the major triggers digestive problems, with one major exception—how stress and psychological factors relate to digestive problems. This is covered next in Chap. 7.

Further Reading

Dysbiosis: gut imbalance, IBD, and more (webmd.com).
Role of the gut microbiota in nutrition and health. PubMed (nih.gov).
The innate and adaptive immune systems. InformedHealth.org. NCBI Bookshelf (nih.gov).
Unhealthy lifestyle and gut dysbiosis: a better understanding of the effects of poor diet and nicotine on the intestinal microbiome. PubMed (nih.gov).

Chapter 7
The Role of Stress and Psychological Factors

A Disclaimer on Stress, Psychological Factors, and Functional Disorders

In Chap. 1, I discussed the difference between "functional" and "organic" gastrointestinal (GI) disorders. This dichotomy is important here because whereas organic disorders can be diagnosed based on tests such as bloodwork, scans, or endoscopy, functional disorders typically cannot be. Thus, in large part because of the absence of abnormal test results, there is a temptation among healthcare providers to be dismissive of functional disorders. Many times, they are chalked up to "just" stress or psychological factors. Sure, either or both of these can be at play and may have a sizable role; however, recent advancements in the understanding of the neurobiology of stress and brain-GI interactions have (1) highlighted the need to appreciate the legitimacy of functional disorders and (2) the importance of stress and psychological factors in both functional as well as organic GI disorders. With all this said, the following tenets should be kept in mind as a disclaimer:

- Having stress or psychological factors present doesn't automatically mean that your digestive problem is "all in your head"; neither does it confine your problem to being strictly a functional disorder.
- Functional disorders can mimic organic disorders, and the converse is true as well. A clinical evaluation, with appropriate testing, is needed to clarify the scenario and diagnosis.
- Even *organic* disorders can be impacted by stress and psychological factors; this and the next tenet are depicted in Fig. 7.1.
- You may have both a functional and an organic disorder; the two are not mutually exclusive, and one isn't necessarily more important than the other.
- Digestive problems can in turn cause or worsen existing stress or psychological problems, hence the bi-directional nature of the relationship.

J. H. Tabibian, *Digestive Problems Solved*, https://doi.org/10.1007/978-3-031-16317-3_7

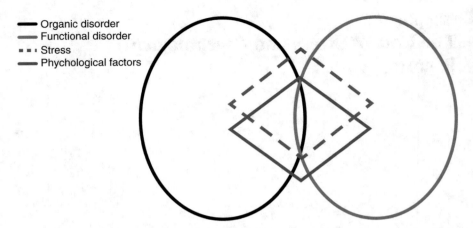

Fig. 7.1 The different combinations that can be seen when thinking about organic GI disorders, functional GI disorders, stress, and psychological factors.
Legend: A given individual may have one, two, three, or all four elements (overlaps are drawn to an arbitrary scale and depend on the disorders being considered and the individual); all elements are important to recognize and appropriateely treat

Stress **and Digestive Problems**

Stress can trigger a whole host of digestive problems including bloating, loss of appetite, increased appetite, constipation, diarrhea, nausea, throat tightness, and more. I can honestly say that I've had first-hand experience with some of these at one point or another. Stress can cause or worsen existing digestive problems. How does this happen, you might ask? Well, the brain and the GI system are intricately connected and constantly in communication, and stress can be seen as a vehicle traveling up and down the connecting freeway between the two. Parenthetically, more neurons, or nerve cells, reside in the GI system than in the entire spinal cord, believe it or not. The effect of stress is also not limited to digestive problems; it's fairly common knowledge, and has been shown in research studies, that stress can cause other problems and symptoms, including headache, a heavy feeling in the chest, fatigue, anxiousness, and so forth. Now throw on top of this personality or mood considerations, which I will discuss in the next section of this chapter, and it becomes quite complicated (some would say even convoluted!).

If the previous paragraph introduced you to some new ideas, that's okay. There is a lot to think about here, and believe it or not, a lot that modern biomedical science doesn't quite understand. For instance, we don't have a clear answer for the simple question: "How exactly does stress cause or worsen digestive problems?" A prevailing theory is that it's due to activation of the "fight-or-flight" response, also known as the sympathetic nervous system. When this response becomes activated, many of our body systems, including GI, may stop functioning normally to help you survive or overcome the stressor as an evolutionary mechanism. For example, if your fight-or-flight response is activated because you're being chased by a lion, don't expect your appetite to be normal or for digestion to function at the same rate as normal—your body is busy prioritizing your survival. What's more, the brain doesn't necessarily know if the stress you're feeling is from being chased by a lion or from some other more commonplace stressor, like a parking ticket, relationship turbulence, financial strain, or work dissatisfaction. All these sources of stress can manifest in the GI system with new or worsened digestive problems.

What to Do about Stress?

First, it's important to be mindful of stress and recognize (i.e. don't deny or be ashamed of) the effects it can have on our GI system and overall health. Second, the importance of stress management should be highlighted. This can take on many different forms. For me, exercise has been extremely useful over the years; controlled physical exertion brings calm of the mind, among many other benefits, which I will discuss in Chap. 12. Numerous other options exist for stress management and can be pursued in combination; these include engaging in yoga, acupuncture, or seeing a therapist, among others, as discussed further in Chap. 14.

Psychological Factors **and Digestive Problems**

Though I'm covering psychological factors (a phrase which I use in a broad sense) in a section separate from stress, many parallels and overlaps exist between the two. This is partly because there is a known dynamic and important interaction between psychology and stress. There's even a method based on their interaction and their partial inseparability: the psychosocial approach. In the psychosocial approach, individuals are studied in the context of the combined influence that psychological factors and the surrounding social environment have on their physical and mental wellness and their ability to function. Remember that we are not living in a vacuum; instead there is constant crosstalk between many factors and components: our GI system, our brain, stressors around us, emotions we feel, etc.

As a gastroenterologist, I try to identify and think about psychological factors in a practical manner so that I can efficiently help patients. I use a framework consisting of three components:

- **History of adverse life events**: These include trauma, sexual abuse, and other major negative events. Having a history of adverse life events is important in the context of digestive problems in two main ways: it can (1) make it more likely that an individual will develop a digestive problem, in particular a functional GI disorder, and (2) influence how an individual feels and deals with a digestive problem, regardless of whether it is a functional or an organic GI disorder. In other words, a history of adverse life events can predispose you to having a digestive problem, in addition to making your experience with one worse. As an example, individuals with irritable bowel syndrome are more likely to have a history of adverse life events than the general population, and they also report more pain, greater psychological distress, and poorer daily function.

- **Mood and other mental health disorders**: These include but are not limited to anxiety, depression, and demoralization. Mood and other mental health disorders are factors that can greatly modify the experience with a digestive problem and, conversely, can develop or worsen consequent to a digestive problem. Imagine that you suffer from anxiety; if you now also are noticing a change in your bowel habits, you may be more inclined to worry excessively about this and assume the worst. Similarly, if you have depression and now also are feeling pain in your abdomen, this can be overwhelming and make your depression even more diffi-cult to manage. Or if you have depression and it causes you to experience nausea and/or loss of appetite, these may not go away until your depression is adequately treated, as they are a manifestation of the depression rather than a primary diges-tive problem. As an aside, it is important to bear in mind here that medications taken for disorders such as anxiety and depression can *cause* a variety of diges-tive problems such as constipation, diahrrea, nausea, and so forth. It's therefore important to review one's medications for potential offending agents.

- **Coping and support**: Like the above two components, how you cope and the amount of support you have can influence how likely you are to develop a diges-tive problem, how strong its effects may be, and how resilient you are. A history of adverse life events and mood and other mental health disorders can both con-tribute to decreased coping skills and decreased access to and/or perception of support. As a gastroenterologist, there may not be a whole lot I can do to help other than provide empathy and advice (in addition to referring to a social worker and/or mental health professional), but just thinking about the importance of coping and support and voicing that these are factors that impact a person's expe-rience with a digestive problem can be valuable and empowering for patients.

What to Do about Psychological Factors?

As with stress, it's important to be mindful of psychological factors, not dismiss their role in the context of GI and overall health, and actually provide an interven-tion for them to minimize their negative impact on digestive problems. An interven-tion could be a referral to a therapist, psychologist, and/or psychiatrist, for example, or trialing a medication used to treat a mental health disorder. There are many options out there, as covered in **Part IV** of this book—typically the rate-limiting step is realizing the importance of psychological factors in the context of digestive problems, including both functional and organic GI disorders.

Putting it all Together

Stress and psychological factors are often overlooked or underestimated in the context of digestive problems. However, they are bi-directionally interconnected with digestive problems and can play an important role in a vast number of digestive problems and in a number of ways, depending on the person and the problem. Stress and psychological issues are ubiquitous, and it is essential to recognize that they can make digestive problems more likely, more severe, or harder to treat; conversely, digestive problems can trigger more stress or certain psychological issues. Sometimes it can even be difficult to know which is the chicken and which is the egg, so to speak. The bottom line is, if stress and psychological factors are playing a role in your digestive problem (something you or your healthcare provider should at least be considering as a possibility), this needs to be appreciated and addressed in order to really take an effective comprehensive approach, and fortunately there are many options for doing so. Next, **Part III** of the book will explore various critical aspects of the medical evaluation and diagnosis of digestive problems, starting with Chap. 8, which covers how to effectively navigate the path to seeing a subspecialist, in particular a gastroenterologist.

Further Reading

Health status by gastrointestinal diagnosis and abuse history. PubMed (nih.gov).
Stress and the sensitive gut. Harvard Health Publishing. Harvard Health.
The gut-brain connection. Harvard Health.
The neurobiology of stress and gastrointestinal disease. Gut (bmj.com).
The role of psychosocial factors in gastrointestinal disorders. Gut (bmj.com).

Part III
Medical Evaluation and Diagnosis: Pearls, Pitfalls, and What I Wish I Knew Sooner

Chapter 8
Effectively Navigating the Path to Seeing a Subspecialist

An Overview of "Referrals"

What Is a "Referral", and What Purpose Does it Serve?

In the context of medicine, a "referral" is a request from a healthcare professional for a consultation or procedure to be rendered by another provider, often one from a different specialty, to the patient being referred. A referral may come in the form of a phone call, fax, email, electronic medical record message or order, eConsult, or other means. Referrals are commonly how a patient comes to the attention of a gastroenterologist or other subspecialist. An example of a basic referral for gastroenterology services would be a fax from a family medicine doctor's office to a gastroenterologist's office stating that the patient is noticing blood in the stool with wiping and that a colonoscopy is being requested. Upon receipt of a referral, the ball would be in the gastroenterologist's court, as discussed later on in this chapter, to take further action.

Due to health insurance or other reasons, a referral from a medical professional is often required prior to rendering of gastroenterology services. Sometimes, however, patients might reach out and directly establish contact with a gastroenterologist if paying cash for services or if insurance permits, also known as "self-refer". While a self-refer may be necessary in some cases, I would say it is generally not advised to bypass being referred by another healthcare provider. It is important to have a trusty (primary care) provider to help coordinate logistics and steer the ship. In addition, not all abdominal symptoms are due to a digestive problem, so directly seeking out a gastroenterologist may actually be misguided (something a primary care provider may be able to recognize from the outset).

The original version of the chapter has been revised. A correction to this chapter can be found at https://doi.org/10.1007/978-3-031-16317-3_15

J. H. Tabibian, *Digestive Problems Solved*, https://doi.org/10.1007/978-3-031-16317-3_8

Who Makes Referrals to Gastroenterology, and Why Does this Matter?

Referrals to gastroenterology can come from a number of referring providers and from a broad array of healthcare settings. To name just a few examples, they may come from an internist, gynecologist, general surgeon, or rheumatologist seeing patients in the office; a nurse practitioner working in an urgent care; a hospitalist doing rounds on inpatients; or a dentist who notices issues that may be related to a digestive problem. In large part because of this, as well as variation among providers of a given speciality, the quality of referrals can be very heterogeneous; some are great, some are ok, and some are low-quality. This is important because the nature of the referral can help facilitate and guide its outcome, as discussed in the next subsection.

Steps after a Referral Is Received

Once a referral is made, it leads to a response on the part of the receiving healthcare provider's team, be it acceptance, a dialogue for clarification purposes, or denial. In the aforementioned example of a patient noticing blood in the stool with wiping, the response may take the form of an appointment made to see the gastroenterologist, questions about whether or not the patient has ever had a colonoscopy, or stating that the patient is out of network and therefore cannot be seen, among other outcomes.

The Nature and Quality of a Referral

As a mechanism for seeing a gastroenterologist, a referral possesses the power to pave (or not) a smooth and effective transition to subspecialty care. While there are many components to the "nature" of a referral, as shown in Table 8.1, perhaps as important as any other is its *quality*. In this context, a high-quality referral would be accurate, concise, *and* comprehensive. It would allow the receiving provider to effectively understand the scenario and thus would be more likely to result in a high-quality outcome, be it a timely consultation, checking important blood tests in advance, ordering a necessary CT scan, coordinating the appropriate set of endoscopic procedures, or a combination of these things.

Table 8.1 Elements to consider with regard to the nature of a medical referral: not all referrals are created equal

Element	Examples of possibilities
Route	Phone call, fax, email, electronic medical record message or order, eConsult
Referring provider specialty	General Internal Medicine, Family Medicine, Emergency Medicine, General Surgery, Gynecology, Dermatology, Dentistry, etc.
Referral source (location/setting)	Clinic, Urgent Care, Emergency Department, Hospital
Level of detail	Low, intermediate, high
Accuracy	Inaccurate, accurate but incomplete, accurate and complete
Scope and breadth	Superficial/elementary, comprehensive with background aspects
Provision of outside records/data	Not included, included in part, all relevant material provided

The Low-quality Referral: Where Gaps Can Potentially Emerge

Too many times, a potentially important digestive problem may be put on the back-burner or otherwise not appropriately addressed by a gastroenterologist due to how the referral request was presented and subsequently interpreted. A referral need not be lengthy or verbose to be high-quality. Even if brief, if it is organized, clear, and containing the requisite relevant information (as we are supposed to learn in medical training), that should do the trick. When a referral falls short of this, it opens the possibilities to gaps in healthcare and suboptimal outcomes. Sometimes, with extra effort and initiative on the part of the receiving specialist provider, the shortcomings of a low-quality referral can be overcome, but this should not be assumed.

Just imagine that a contestant on "Who Wants to be a Millionaire?" leverages the "Phone a friend" option but words the question in a way that is unclear or inadvertently misleading; chances are the correct response will not be given; the same can happen with a referral. Just as initiating the call to "Phone a friend" is not, in and of itself, sufficient to come up with the correct response, making a referral requires thoughtfulness and diligence to help ensure the proper outcome.

The Referring Provider as the Hub

The referring provider can really be an essential hub in the completion of a medical evaluation, and there are two key interfaces to consider, as illustrated in Fig. 8.1. These two interfaces are between the patient and the referring provider and between the referring provider and specialist.

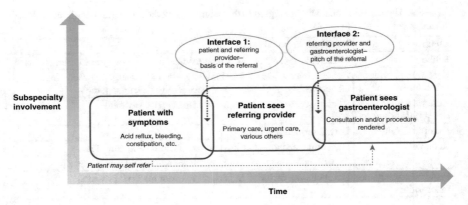

Fig. 8.1 The referring provider as a key central hub in a patient's road to receiving gastroenterology care.
Legend: The general clinical flow with digestive problems is that as time goes on or symptoms become more troublesome, gastroenterology or other subspeciality involvement will typically increase. Of note, a small subset of patients will self-refer for subspecialty care, bypassing interface 1, which may save time up front but may not necessarily be advisable in many cases

Interface Between Patient and the Referring Provider: The Basis of the Referral

So you have a digestive problem, or maybe several. You might wait it out to see if things improve or try things on your own like drinking less coffee or soda, or you may be proactive early on and seek healthcare without delay. When you do decide to seek healthcare, depending on factors such as the nature of your problem, the amount of time you have available to schedule an appointment, your style/preferences, and your available care options, you might first see your primary care provider—who may be a family medicine doctor, an internist, a gynecologist, or other—or you might head to an urgent care or even the emergency department. So, what needs to be achieved and conveyed during this visit with your potential referring provider to-be?

First and foremost, one must of course assess for red flags, such as vomiting blood or unintentional weight loss. As discussed in Chap. 3, these may be indicators of a severe or serious condition and, if present, would dictate a certain approach to expedited referral. Let's assume that red flags are not present, as with most individuals who have digestive problems; perhaps you just have a sour taste in the mouth, heartburn, or occasional loose stools. It is largely your responsibility to adequately express the key facets of your problem(s) and the responsibility of the provider to adequately understand them. Though as a patient it is not possible to completely control what the referring provider will understand and accordingly recommend thereafter, you can certainly do certain things to make the task clearer and more fool-proof. Table 8.2 provides a summary in this regard, which I will expand upon based on the pre-visit, during visit, and post-visit stages.

Table 8.2 The "OLD CARTS" and "WILDA" symptom mnemonics

Mnemonic	Individual components
OLD CARTS	*O*nset
	*L*ocation
	*D*uration
	*C*haracteristics
	*A*ggravating factors
	*R*elieving factors
	*T*reatments
	*S*everity
WILDA	*W*ords to describe
	*I*ntensity
	*L*ocation
	*D*uration
	*A*ggravating/*a*lleviating factors

Legend: Well-prepared patients should be able to furnish this information to their healthcare provider.

Things to Do Pre-Visit

Just as you would do for a job interview or when taking a tour of a university you are considering, you should try to come prepared. This might mean different things to different people. Does it mean you should look up your problem on Google or Wikipedia and try to become an expert? Not necessarily, but you might choose to do some reading or independent learning in order to gain some background knowledge and familiarity. But do not let this come at this expense of paying attention to what exactly you are feeling. At the very least, reflect on and be cognizant of what it is that you are feeling, when you feel it, how long it has been going on for, and so forth. For instance, if you are having pain under your breastbone, is it a burning pain, cramping pain, or stabbing pain? And does it occur all the time, or only after eating tomato sauce, or when you are feeling hungry or in the morning when you first wake up? Has it been there for just two weeks, or for the last 10 years? These are all useful and sometimes highly telling details, and you should have them at the tip of your tongue or written down so as to not forget to relate them.

Some individuals will choose to keep a log or diary of their problem. This can be helpful and informative, but at the same time you do not want to become so bogged down by it that you are obsessing about your problem. Keeping a symptom diary or at least taking some notes can be most important for individuals who otherwise would not be able to answer the questions that healthcare providers will typically ask as part of symptom assessment. These questions include those that comprise medical mnemonics such as those shown in Table 8.2.

Things to Do during the Visit

This is your chance to impress upon the to-be referring provider what you are experiencing. The visit can sometimes be overwhelming, with finding parking, not feeling well, a long wait in the lobby, and so on, but the preparatory elements mentioned in the preceding paragraph will help mitigate this. In addition to being ready to relate your problem, also be prepared to answer questions about your past medical history and family history; you never know when these could tie into what you have going on.

Also, recognize that it is possible for the referring provider, not just the patient, to become overwhelmed. For example, the provider can become overwhelmed when patients go on and on talking without checking in with the provider (making eye contact, for instance) to see if they are on the same page. So while you want to be detailed and accurate in what you share, you also want to be succinct and take periodic breaks to make sure your provider is following along. On a related note, if you have medical records to bring, try to just bring what seems pertinent rather than a big pile of papers. It is also helpful if the records are organized and that any color photos are actually in color, if possible. Furthermore, do not assume that the provider has had time to read everything about you ahead of time. Lastly, try to avoid vague explanation such as "for a while" or "in my stomach." The more methodical you can be in this regard, the more you help the referring provider direct your care, including the referral, in the right direction.

Interface Between the Referring Provider and Subspecialist: The Pitch of the Referral

After you see the referring provider and assuming they are not able to independently address the problem you have, a referral will be placed for gastroenterology or other subspecialty evaluation. This is a critical interface, but how exactly the process unfolds can be enigmatic for insurance and other reasons. However, there are things you can do as the patient or caregiver as part of diligent follow up and being one's own best advocate.

As you Await the Subspecialist Visit

If you are contacted by the gastroenterologist's office promptly, that's generally a good sign. It is when you have *not* been contacted promptly that you might need to become involved. It is ok to ask the referring provider's office questions, like "Was the office able to send the referral?" or "Which gastroenterologist's office did the staff send the referral to?" or "Do you know if my recent abnormal test results were included in the referral so the gastroenterologist can appreciate the relative urgency?" Alternatively, if your referring provider has an electronic health record system with a patient portal, you can look to see what information was conveyed and what type of referral request was made. Such a portal can be a useful avenue for doing your part to ensure your referral is going through as expected. If you know to which gastroenterologist you have been referred, you can also reach out to that office to check on the status of your referral, if there are any particular records or other materials they would like you to bring, and so forth.

Unfortunately, sometimes referrals leave out important information, can be accepted later than what is ideal, or result in an appointment that is scheduled far out. If you have the sense that this may be the case, it is your right to become involved to help expedite the proper evaluation and care, and you have various options as far as how to go about doing so.

When Time Comes to See the Subspecialist

In the interest of not being redundant, all of the tenets and principles presented in the paragraphs above regarding how to best ensure an effective visit with the referring provider also apply to your visit with the gastroenterologist. In brief, be prepared to tell your story, stay focused and clear, try to be accurate with the details, and avoid assuming that the gastroenterologist already knows every piece of information about your case. Do not be surprised if the gastroenterologist goes into greater detail than what is covered by the mnemonics in Table 8.2, at least with certain questions. For example, the gastroenterologist may inquire about what time of day the problem occurs, if it correlates with certain meals or foods, how long it lasts when it comes on, if it ever wakes you up from sleep, if it radiates to another part of your body, what you have done to try to alleviate it, or whether it has changed at all since you saw the referring provider. If you do not know something, it is quite okay to say so.

Putting it all Together

The most common route for a patient to see a gastroenterologist is through a referral. A referral is essentially a professional request that is typically placed by a primary care provider, though it could come from other healthcare providers and from a variety of healthcare settings. There are considerable differences among referring providers and the referrals they make; some referrals are higher quality than others, and the higher the quality, the more likely a referral will be handled appropriately for your digestive problem. While you cannot fully control how a referral is made, there are a number of steps you can take as a patient or caregiver to make the right impression on the referring provider and equip her/him with relevant and sufficient information. Many of these steps are not only useful for your encounter with the referring provider, but also in turn for your encounter with the gastroenterologist. Indeed, they can help you to become a solid advocate and all the more efficiently get to the bottom of your digestive problem. One specific benefit in this regard is that they will also more effectively inform your healthcare provider with regard to the medical testing you may need, as will be covered next in Chap. 9.

Further Reading

https://www.aafp.org/pubs/afp/issues/2012/0201/p279.html
https://www.acponline.org/clinical-information/high-value-care/resources-for-clinicians/
   high-value-care-coordination-hvcc-toolkit

Chapter 9
Following a Practical Sequence in Testing

Components and Sequence of the Medical Diagnostic Evalution

As healthcare providers learn during their education and training, there are certain components that constitute a diagnostic medical evaluation. These should generally follow a certain sequence, whether the provider is a general internist, gastroenterologist, or other (Fig. 9.1), and can be summarized as follows:

- Consultation: The initial consultation between a healthcare provider and patient includes multiple elements, including the history of present illness, review of symptoms, medications, family history, and physical examination. All of these are important, and any one of them could hold the key to what is going on, so it's essential to lay a sound foundation here. As discussed in Chap. 8, it is typical to ask detailed questions about the symptom(s). This helps to paint a clear picture of what is going on, construct a list of possible diagnoses, also called a "differential diagnosis", and map out next steps. The differential diagnosis is a fundamental aspect of medicine and is a reflection of one's clinical judgment and breadth of knowledge. If, for example, a provider does not think to include problem x in the differential diagnosis, then it is likely that testing for it will not occur and that the diagnosis will be missed or delayed, leading to lost time, additional costs, and patient frustration and morbidity.
- Laboratory testing: This includes testing of blood, urine, stool, breath, and other specimen types. The specimen type and what exactly is tested for are guided based on the differential diagnosis. If a patient presents with diarrhea, as you may imagine, we would want to test the stool. But there are also a number of blood tests that can shed light on certain causes of diarrhea, such as endocrine causes, that the stool may or may not shed light on. Thus, the differential diagnosis provides a crucial roadmap for testing.

J. H. Tabibian, *Digestive Problems Solved*,
https://doi.org/10.1007/978-3-031-16317-3_9

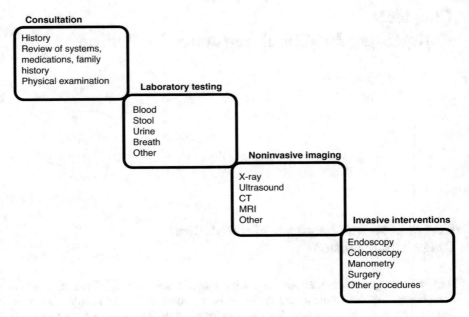

Fig. 9.1 Components and sequence of the diagnostic evaluation.
Legend: Shown here is an overview of the general components of the diagnostic evaluation and
the sequence in which they would typically take place, from top left to bottom right. This list is not
exhaustive, and a diagnosis can be achieved in some cases without having to complete all four
components of the evaluation

- Noninvasive imaging: This consists of things like X-rays, ultrasounds, CT scans,
  and MRIs, among other imaging modalities, or types. They provide a look inside
  the body and are considered noninvasive since nothing is being put in the body
  aside perhaps from contrast, which some of these modalities may utilize. Contrast
  can be oral, intravenous, or other, and helps make a given imaging modality more
  sensitive and higher yield. One example of contrast would be barium that is swallowed as part of a swallowing assessment known as a barium esophagram. Some
  contrast agents can be harmful though, hence they need to be used with caution
  and conscientiously. Each imaging modality also has its relative strengths and
  weaknesses. This is critically important; I will sometimes see patients who have
  had a certain scan, say an abdominal ultrasound, and it is "negative" or "normal".
  This is great, but ultrasound is not useful for looking at hollow or air-filled
  organs, such as the stomach or intestines. Therefore, a negative ultrasound provides only a finite amount of reassurance and is certainly not the end of the search.
- Invasive interventions: These include things like endoscopy, colonoscopy, esophageal and anorectal manometry, and surgery, among others. Invasive interventions can be diagnostic or therapeutic, and sometimes they are both, as noted here:

    - Diagnostic: Used to make a diagnosis. Imagine a patient who is thought to
      have inflammation of the esophagus, or esophagitis, based on symptoms but

the healthcare provider is still not sure. An upper endoscopy may be performed to take a better look and establish a diagnosis.
- Therapeutic: Used to treat a problem. Imagine a similar patient, but in this case a noninvasive imaging study shows a benign-appearing esophageal stricture, or abnormal narrowing. An upper endoscopy would be performed to open up the stricture using a dilation balloon or other instrument.
- Both diagnostic and therapeutic: Used both to make a diagnosis and treat a problem. Imagine another similar patient, but in this case a noninvasive test shows a malignant-appearing mass blocking the esophagus. An upper endoscopy could be performed both to obtain biopsies of the mass (diagnostic) as well as to place a stent as a treatment to open up the esophagus so that food can pass through when the patient eats (therapeutic).

Some patients or providers will not want to follow this sequence in testing, instead wanting to skip ahead, but most will be amenable to it. Each component can inform the next and make the next more purposeful and efficient. Moreover, there are times when you won't even know that a subsequent step is needed until you perform the preceding, more fundamental tests. In many if not most cases, patience and adherence to this general sequence is advisable.

When Is (Further) Testing Needed?

Sometimes a healthcare provider can confidently determine what digestive problem a patient has just based on obtaining a careful history. Other times, either the obtained history is not comprehensive enough or more information is needed beyond what can be discerned from the initial consultation. In such instances, there is a need to progress down the list of components of the diagnostic evaluation. There are also times where the healthcare provider probably knows what is going on, but further testing is needed to either confirm it or to rule out other similar conditions. Keep in mind, however, that more testing can also lead to more costs and sometimes detect inconsequential normal variants that lead to more worry, and in turn further testing; the expression "chasing one's tail" has been used in this scenario. As an example, picture that you are taking your car in to get checked out for a loud-sounding exhaust. The experienced technician may know that the issue is your muffler simply based on how it sounds; so do you want to go ahead and resolve the muffler issue, or do you prefer the technician charge you for additional tests that may not be needed and might even lead to recommendations to make unnecessary repairs? Thus, more testing isn't always better.

Fortunately, there are various clinical practice guidelines from a number of gastroenterological and other professional societies which lay out recommended approaches to not only diagnostic testing but also, treatment, screening, and other aspects of care for a wide range of digestive problems. These may be regarded as the standard of care and are often the best way of going about managing digestive problems. These guidelines aren't hard and fast rules, however, and individualized deviations may occur, as each individual scenario is different. Whenever possible, I usually like to combine what is outlined in clinical practice guidelines with what the individual needs and wishes of a given patient may be. Take for example a 40-year-old patient who presents with typical features of gastroesophageal reflux disease (GERD). The patient reports 5 years of intermittent GERD that has worsened in the last 6 months, in association with weight gain. Practice guidelines would likely recommend starting acid suppression therapy and assessing the response in approximately 8 weeks. In other words, there is no clear need to order laboratory tests, non-invasive imaging, or endoscopy at this juncture. But what if these symptoms are causing the patient substantial emotional distress because they had an uncle who died of some kind of "throat" cancer? Here, I would say there is an individualized justification to pursue some form of further testing, both for peace of mind and also to make sure that the worsening "GERD" isn't a red herring that is masking an underlying sinister esophageal problem, such as esophageal cancer.

Instances Where the Usual Testing Sequence May Not Be Best

There are many instances wherein a step-by-step sequence may be bypassed. In emergency scenarios, there may not be time to follow a stepwise sequence of evaluation components, and instead an invasive intervention is needed right away. Even in these scenarios, though, certain algorithms tend to be followed. For example, someone walking in with chest pain does not go straight to an angiogram or open heart surgery; a basic history will typically be obtained, followed by vital signs, cardiac enzyme levels in the blood, an ECG, chest x-ray, and other tests and measures, which might then be followed by an invasive intervention. In the context of digestive problems, there are a number of scenarios wherein at the end of the day, an endoscopic procedure such as an upper endoscopy or colonoscopy will most likely be needed regardless of what preceding tests or noninvasive imaging may show. In these scenarios, it is reasonable to go ahead and move forward with the endoscopic procedure.

Imagine for instance a 55-year-old who has been noticing blood in her stool for the last month, but otherwise feels fine. A stool test to check for microscopic blood probably isn't necessary since the patient is seeing blood with his naked eye. Plus, if the stool test comes back negative, would that nullify the need for further evaluation? Similarly, an X-ray of the abdomen would probably not be needed in this case since it is highly unlikely that it would change the fact that something needs to be done about the visible blood in the stool. This is a scenario wherein the patient should go ahead and undergo a diagnostic colonoscopy to ascertain what the source of the bleeding is. I will say that sometimes having blood tests done beforehand can be useful to gauge the safety of an endoscopic procedure, and similarly noninvasive imaging beforehand can provide a useful roadmap for an endoscopic procedure (granted it does not delay the time to procedure); these are decisions that can be made as appropriate on a case-by-case basis.

A Few Words on Endoscopy

As a gastroenterologist, I would be remiss if I did not have at least a brief section regarding endoscopic procedures. In the most fundamental sense, endoscopy refers to looking inside the body, typically the digestive tract. It is achieved using an endoscope, which is essentially a thin, flexible tube with a light, a camera, and usually a channel through which instruments, such as a biopsy forceps, can be pased. The endoscope is inserted through the mouth for upper endoscopy or through the anus for colonoscopy. There are various types of endoscopes for various types of endoscopic procedures; for example, a gastroscope used for upper endoscopy is smaller in diameter and shorter in length than a colonoscope used for colonoscopy. Most endoscopic procedures are brief, lasting approximately 10–30 min, but some can be much longer. Some form of sedation is usually provided for both patient comfort and safety, the type sedation depending on the individual patient and the planned procedure.

When performed by an experienced team, endoscopic procedures are generally very safe. Minor adverse events, such as a sore throat following upper endoscopy or bloating following a colonoscopy, may occur but typically are mild. There is a small risk of serious adverse events such as perforation or severe bleeding, but fortunately these are very rare. Despite its general safety, I would say endoscopy should still be taken seriously and pursued only if there is a sound indication for it. Not everyone with a digestive problem needs an endoscopy; however, after following a stepwise sequence in their diagnostic evaluation, the need for an endoscopy becomes apparent for many patients because it offers the opportunity to directly see what's going on inside the digestive tract and, if necessary, take samples directly from it. As with any intervention, especially an invasive one, it is important to consider the risks, benefits, and alternatives and review these with your healthcare provider. A sound understanding of these as well as the steps needed to prepare for an endoscopic procedure, such as fasting or drinking a bowel purgative solution starting the day prior, are essential. This understanding also helps ease excess anxiety in addition to increasing procedural safety and efficacy.

How Do I Know if My Evaluation Is Complete?

It is difficult to know if your evaluation for a digestive problem is sufficient or complete, as the diagnostic possibilities are vast, and every situation is unique. If you have received the information you sought in the form of a diagnosis and there is an effective plan in place for your treatment—for instance, medication is prescribed, and after a reasonable period of time you are feeling back to normal—then your evaluation is probably sufficient. On the other hand, feeling in the dark, not understanding what's going on, having symptoms that are not improving despite treatment, or lacking a plan in terms of what more needs to be done diagnostically or therapeutically are all indicators that your evaluation may be insufficient or incomplete. Try to be an advocate for yourself and for your GI system; ask questions that are important to you, listen carefully, and try to build a bond with your healthcare provider. Despite your efforts, sometimes it just is not possible to achieve all of these, or your digestive problem may not be appropriately evaluated for some other reason. In Chap. 11, we will discuss scenarios where seeking out a second opinion may be in your best interest.

Putting it all Together

There are several components to the diagnostic medical evaluation. This first component, i.e. the consultation, sets the stage for subsequent components, such as laboratory testing, noninvasive imaging, or invasive interventions. Some patients will need to complete all of the components, whereas in other cases, a diagnosis may be reached through the initial consultation alone or at some other early point. There are also instances where it may be appropriate to not go through the traditional sequence of components and instead skip ahead, such as to an invasive intervention like endoscopy. What makes an evaluation sufficiently comprehensive depends on the individual and their digestive problem, as each case is different. Some cases are relatively straightforward and simple to evaluate, diagnose, and accordingly treat, whereas others may require quite a bit of investigation or even a second opinion. In this chapter, we discussed the notion of the differential diagnosis as being an integral piece of a medical evaluation. Next, in Chap. 10, we will discuss a related concept, that of the "unifying diagnosis".

Further Reading

ASGE. Practice guidelines—standards of practice.
Efficient diagnostic test sequence: applications of the probability-modifying plot. PubMed (nih.gov).
Endoscopy. NHS (www.nhs.uk).
Guidelines. American College of Gastroenterology (gi.org).
Guidelines. American Gastroenterological Association.
Malpractice comparative benchmarking system reports (harvard.edu).
Practice guidelines. AASLD.
The diagnostic process: rediscovering the basic steps (thesullivangroup.com).
Upper GI endoscopy. NIDDK (nih.gov).

Chapter 10
The Unifying Diagnosis: Often but Not Always Correct

Basis of the Unifying Diagnosis

Difficulties in making a diagnosis occur in all areas of healthcare yet need to be overcome in order to optimally treat and manage patients. Digestive problems are no exception to this. The difficulties can stem from various sources. For example:

- There may be no apparent (cognitive) match between a provider's assessment of a problem and a specific diagnosis,
- The correct diagnosis may be clouded by confounding factors or by atypical presenting features, or
- There may be compelling evidence of more than one diagnosis being present.

To help effectively navigate these difficulties, we are taught as healthcare professionals to look for a unifying diagnosis that could explain all of the patient's presenting symptoms rather than providing several explanations for them. The notion of the unifying diagnosis dates back to William of Ockham, a Franciscan monk in the early fourteenth century who studied at the Universities of Oxford and Paris. He is credited for having written "*Numquam ponenda est pluralitas sine necessitate*," which can be translated as "*Plurality ought never be posed without necessity.*" This line of thought has been termed "Ockham's Razor", which is the principle that, when presented with competing explanations, the simplest explanation is usually the best one, as exemplified in Fig. 10.1. In medicine, what this suggests is that the simplest (or most "parsimonious") explanation for any given set of symptoms is most likely to be correct. Consider, for example, two cases:

1. A 30-year-old woman presents with several months of fluctuations in stool appearance and frequency as well as bloating-type abdominal pain that improves after defecation. In order to account for these symptoms, a plurality-based approach might lead the provider to believe that this patient has an intestinal parasite, a partial bowel obstruction, and maybe even Celiac disease

© The Author(s), under exclusive license to Springer Nature Switzerland AG 2023
J. H. Tabibian, *Digestive Problems Solved*,
https://doi.org/10.1007/978-3-031-16317-3_10

Plurality-based explanation:	Problem: A tree has fallen down. Why?	Unifying diagnosis explanation:
There were two meteorites involved. The first one came down and struck the tree, knocking it over. The second one then struck the first one, and both turned to dust, thereby leaving no evidence behind.		The wind knocked the tree down.

Fig. 10.1 Solving a problem with a plurality-based approach vs. a unifying diagnosis approach. **Legend:** Ockham's razor favors a single explanation (i.e. a "unifying diagnosis") rather than one that is complex and entails unnecessary assumptions. The former is more likely to be correct in a majority of cases

or inflammatory bowel disease (IBD). A unifying diagnosis approach, however, can successfully diagnose this patient with irritable bowel syndrome (IBS). Assuming no findings that argue against a diagnosis of IBS, this would be the most practical and accurate explanation for the patient's stool changes and abdominal pain. This correct unifying diagnosis is important, as it opens a window to focused testing and appropriate therapeutic intervention rather than chasing multiple inaccurate explanations.

2. A 40-year-old man presents with burning under his sternum, a bitter taste in his mouth in the mornings, and recent weight gain. A plurality-based approach might lead the provider to believe that this patient has a pneumonia or heart problem, lead poisoning, and a thyroid tumor that is causing him to gain weight. A unifying diagnosis approach, however, may successfully diagnose this patient with gastroesophageal reflux disease (GERD), which may well have surfaced due to the recent weight gain. The extra weight in the abdominal area could push on his stomach and cause reflux of acidic, bitter-tasting gastric juices into the esophagus and throat. It would be far more efficient to manage the GERD in this case rather than chase multiple independent (and erroneous) diagnoses.

Problems with the Unifying Diagnosis

Although trying to find a unifying diagnosis is justifiable and desirable from a philosophy of medicine standpoint, in some cases it does not exist. As healthcare providers, we need to consider all possible diagnoses for a given patient presentation and try to come up with a unifying diagnosis while also being open to the possibility that multiple diagnoses may truly be present. I will use the same two examples from above, modified slightly to illustrate problems with the unifying diagnosis:

1. Picture the same 30-year-old woman from above, but in addition, she states she has seen blood in her stool. Blood in stool is not a feature of IBS. Therefore, either IBS is not actually the correct unifying diagnosis, or it is not the *only* diag-

nosis. I've seen both of these scenarios happen: in the first scenario, what was thought to be IBS was actually IBD or early-onset colorectal cancer whereas in the second scenario, the patient did in fact meet diagnostic criteria for IBS but also had internal hemorrhoids, a common cause of rectal bleeding.

2. Picture the same 40-year-old man from above, but in addition, he reports vomiting. Like the preceding example, vomiting is not a feature of GERD. Thus, either GERD is not the correct unifying diagnosis, or it is not the *only* diagnosis. As with the first example, I've seen both of these scenarios happen: in the first scenario, what was thought to be GERD was actually a disease known as "achalasia", whereas in the second scenario, the patient did actually have GERD, but there was also an esophageal stricture, a known complication of longstanding GERD in a subset of patients.

The Unifying Diagnosis: Use Only if it Fits

Ultimately, despite the merits of the unifying diagnosis, there are potential hazards with it and its associated biases. The major one is the possibility of becoming absorbed with a single explanation for a set of symptoms and not taking a step back to consider alternative or additional diagnoses. It is important to recognize that just because a patient has a set of symptoms attributable to digestive problem X doesn't mean that problem Y isn't also lurking behind the scenes. Providers have to be willing to entertain such possibilities and be astute and vigilant, especially if a patient's symptoms evolve over time. Changes may indicate either that problem X has progressed or that problem Y has now also developed. Therefore, if you've been given a diagnosis for your digestive problem but have persistent symptoms without clear answers or direction, or if your diagnosis doesn't seem to fit well, you and your healthcare provider should be thinking about alternative explanations and considering additional evaluation.

Putting it all Together

Thinking of and making the correct diagnosis can be a challenging task, but it is essential to coming up with the right care plan. Otherwise, an off-target diagnosis can lead to off-course clinical management, which tends to be ineffective and can even be unsafe. As healthcare providers, we learn about clinical parsimony and the related concept of the "unifying diagnosis." The unifying diagnosis is frequently helpful and correct but not always careful; medical evaluation and critical thinking are needed on an individualized basis. An initial diagnosis can of course be incorrect, so an open mind and sharp eye are necessary, and at times further evaluation is needed. In some cases, a second opinion is advisable, and that is the topic covered next in Chap. 11.

Further Reading

Cognitive bias in clinical medicine. PubMed (nih.gov).
Ockham's razor: sharpen or re-sheathe? PubMed (nih.gov).
The unifying diagnosis. PubMed (nih.gov).

Chapter 11
Seeking a Second Opinion: When and Where

Should I Obtain a Second Opinion?

Whether or not you should obtain a second opinion is a complex and personal matter that depends on the perceived benefits and drawbacks. As you think this question through (Fig. 11.1), there are perhaps two fundamental points to keep in mind:

1. If you are feeling uneasiness with your healthcare or it is not resonating with you, it is likely you will gain from a second opinion. Maybe the second opinion will bring with it a perspective that resonates better with your views and wishes.
2. What you ultimately walk away with from a second opinion will not always be what you expected from the outset. Sometimes there are surprises, more often positive than not, to second opinions.

The Benefits of a Second Opinion

A few benefits to obtaining a second opinion would be:

- To confirm what you already know/have been told
- To learn more about your problem or feel more comfortable about it
- To have peace of mind knowing that you have done everything you can to ensure that you have the correct information and plan moving forward
- To gain insights into options, whether diagnostic or therapeutic, that may not have been previously mentioned
- To narrow down choices and help make a decision

Some patients might identify more with one benefit than the other, while a handful of patients will identify with several of these benefits.

J. H. Tabibian, *Digestive Problems Solved*,
https://doi.org/10.1007/978-3-031-16317-3_11

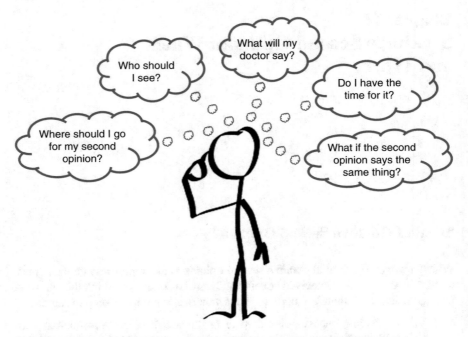

Fig. 11.1 Questions that arise when thinking about obtaining a second opinion

Situations that Merit a Second Opinion

Broadly speaking, I would suggest that a patient with a digestive problem seek, or at least consider, a second opinion if any of these apply:

- *You are undergoing or have undergone treatment but your symptoms persist.* Perhaps the treatment is not working because the diagnosis is not correct or the treatment is not the right choice for you; this needs to be looked into further. You should go back to your existing healthcare provider, and if your provider is not sure what else to do or says there is nothing more to do, that is usually prime time for a second opinion. Not every provider has the same vantage point, and some may be more knowledgeable about or have more experience with your particular problem than others.
- *The recommended treatment is invasive.* Anytime you are entertaining a recommendation to pursue an invasive intervention, especially a surgery, it is important to evaluate your options thoroughly and think critically. It is your body and life, after all, and you are entitled to playing a central role in your healthcare decisions, especially major decisions. Surgery is likely to be potentially irreversible; being proactive about such an important decision will grant you a greater degree of control over your treatment outcome. I once had surgery while I was in training and did not pursue a second opinion beforehand. I felt confident in my surgeon, was not under the impression that the surgery was all that big, and did not want to waste my or anyone else's time. It was only after I sought a second

opinion post-operation that I realized how much I had missed out on. In truth, this has been one of my major life regrets.

- *You are diagnosed with a rare disease.* Rare diseases, as the name implies, are those that afflict a relatively small number of patients. There are approximately 7000 known rare diseases according to the National Institutes for Health, some of which relate to the gastrointestinal system. Frankly, not everyone can be an expert in every rare disease, even within one's specialty. In fact, chances are that your healthcare provider is not an expert in your particular rare disease (unless you sought them out specifically for it). Granted this is not the case, if your healthcare provider is not suggesting referral to an expert for a second opinion on your problem, you should look into this yourself to benefit from the most up-to-date and accurate information (and who knows, maybe you do not even actually have the rare disease!).

- *You are diagnosed with cancer or other potentially terminal illness.* A diagnosis of cancer is scary on so many levels; it is like your body is betraying itself and turning on you. Though many cancers are curable, some are not, and some are in a gray zone. The first thing to is to be sure that the diagnosis is accurate, so you might seek out a second opinion just for that. Sometimes the diagnosis is very clear, but the devil lies in the details. Unless starting treatment is an emergency, you should consider a second opinion to better gauge the various treatment options available. Moreover, there are sometimes research studies which will give you access to the latest and greatest medicines, but not every healthcare provider is participating in them. Thus, it helps to cast the second opinion net from the outset (as well as down the road if issues arise).

- *Your mind (or gut) tells you something is off.* Some patients have really good instincts, maybe even better than their healthcare providers. The provider may have the advantage of formal medical education and training, but you likely know yourself and your body better. Trust in yourself and do not settle—pause, reflect, talk to your loved ones, and read up on your condition if you feel like something is off with the problem you are experiencing or the care you are receiving. Be an advocate for yourself and ask questions. Sometimes you will need to take a step to broaden your perspectives by obtaining a second opinion; it may open up truly helpful avenues.

Concerns Around Getting a Second Opinion

While obtaining a second opinion can yield additional perspectives that increase the likelihood that you will come away with the best possible care plan and outcomes, it can have some downsides.

- Time: it takes time, and sometimes a lot of it, to look into, arrange, and go to a second opinion. In the moment, it can seem like it is too time-consuming. But in the grand scheme of things, it may be a few hours that can end up serving you for the rest of your life. With more options for virtual visits emerging, a second opinion often need not require as much time as you might think, and especially for serious digestive problems, is probably well worth it.

- Cost: as with time, second opinions can require some investment or cost. Your health insurance policy is probably the main determining factor here. Fortunately, with many insurance carriers, the cost for a second opinion is no greater than for the first opinion, unless the second opinion provider is out-of-network. If out-of-network, an additional copayment may apply. Even so, you should view a second opinion as an investment, and while it is conceivable that in the end you will be no further along than before, many patients gain valuable dividends from a second opinion.
- Feeling of shame or fear of retaliation: it is not uncommon for patients to feel uncomfortable or even ashamed if they request a second opinion. However, second opinions are common and a patient's right, and you should not have to worry about your healthcare provider shaming you, becoming upset, or retaliating in some way. I would be wary of healthcare providers who frown at the notion of a second opinion (or who claim to know it all or to have a panacea); conversely, a confident and thoughtful provider might welcome a second opinion.

While there are some downsides to second opinions, I find that when a second opinion is thought of, more often than not its benefits end up outweighing the downsides.

Where and How to Obtain a Second Opinion

Where and how to obtain a second opinion can depend on a variety of factors, including your particular digestive problem, where you are located, what healthcare providers you have seen so far, what insurance you have, and more. Once you have obtained a second opinion, you have the option of returning to your initial provider or continuing your care with the second opinion provider, or in some instances both. The choice is generally yours, based on your preferences.

Where to Go for a Second Opinion

With regard to where to obtain a second opinion, I often say go to the institution or provider with the most expertise. Analogous to the concept of practice makes perfect, the more a provider has seen patients with your digestive problem, and the more they have a vested interest in that problem, the better they will be at managing it. However, there are times where you may find a diamond in the rough or when you may go to a world-renowned institution but not actually be seen by the most fitting provider, i.e. the expert in your specific digestive problem. The institution or provider with the most expertise may also be across the country, so you may need to balance out expertise with proximity, convenience, and cost. Many times there will be an expert in your region who is, for all practical purposes, as experienced as the expert across the country.

Taking a step back, some individuals may face the issue of not knowing who or where the institution or provider with the most expertise is. In such scenarios, reading up online for publications related to your digestive problem, talking to family and friends, and discussing with your primary care provider or even the first subspecialist you see can prove useful.

How to Go About Obtaining a Second Opinion

There are several potential routes to going about obtaining a second opinion:

- Talk to your primary care provider. If they have not provided you a referral to a subspecialist such as a gastroenterologist, request one. In a sense, if you have not seen a subspecialist yet, then this would not even be a *second* opinion but rather a first. A primary care provider could ostensibly take offense to this, but in my experience, most would welcome the input and help of a subspecialist, especially if you frame it graciously. For example, "I really am appreciative of your attention to this matter. Given how much it is troubling me, and so as to not take up too much of your time, would it be possible to refer me to a subspecialist for some additional perspective and further management?" I have used a similar line myself as a patient, and it has worked quite well. If your primary care provider has already referred you to a subspecialist and you already saw said individual, you can simply ask for the name of an additional provider that they would recommend. They might want to know why you want an additional name, in which case feel free to elaborate.
- If you are already seeing a subspecialist, ask them if there is another subspecialist that they could recommend as someone they would trust to provide a second opinion. Sometimes this can create an uncomfortable situation, as discussed in the previous section. However, second opinions are becoming more and more commonplace as patients are becoming increasingly inquisitive and informed. Do not be deterred—you need to be resolute and determined as your own best advocate. At the same time, just as you would with your primary care provider, you can be gracious with the subspecialist: "I really appreciate the time and thought you have invested in my case. I would like to do everything I can on my end to make a sound decision in this regard, as this is an important decision for me. Is there anyone or anywhere you could perhaps recommend to me for a second opinion? I think this would help provide me some additional perspective and peace of mind."
- Reach out to local or national professional societies, such as the American Gastroenterological Association or American College of Gastroenterology, for names of recommended providers in your area or across the country.
- Do your own research (Google, Google Scholar, PubMed.gov, etc.) on your digestive problem and see who seems to be an authority in the area.

Some patients will pursue several of these routes, and others perhaps just one. Regardless, it may be prudent to discuss with your health insurance carrier, as certain rules or limitations may apply. The other benefit to discussing with the insurance provider is that often times they have a list of in-network providers and can tell you which providers may be associated with additional out-of-network fees.

Digestive Problem Scenarios Where You May Benefit from a Second Opinion

Patients and providers have contacted me on many occasions to provide a second (or third or fourth) opinion on a variety of matters. As such, I thought it would be useful to provide some relatively common digestive problems for which a second opinion may be sought and the ways in which it could help shed light at different junctures in the course of having a problem. Imagine you are:

1. A patient with severe constipation who is not getting better with laxatives.

    (a) Your definition of constipation may not be the medical definition of constipation. For example, some patients think they need to defecate at least once a day to be "regular." That is not really the case; as infrequently as once every 3 days is considered normal, granted you are not having to strain excessively to have a bowel movement.

    (b) If you really are constipated, you may not be taking the right laxative regimen, your dose may be too low, or you may need to give the regimen more time. You should not expect a 180° change in just a day or two, especially for a chronic problem like constipation; expectations need to be appropriately aligned.

    (c) You may have tried several bowel regimens and given them each the proper amount of time to take effect. Before giving up and resorting to potentially drastic measures, you should know that there are some lesser-known prescription medicines that many providers are not familiar with or do not prescribe; these could be tried as a next step.

    (d) You may be taking medications that cause contstipation for which non-constipating alternatives exist. Periodically reviewing your medication list with your healthcare provider as well as a pharmacist is important.

    (e) In rare instances, patients are referred for surgery to remove part of their colon as a treatment for severe constipation that is not responding to an appropriate laxative regimen. However, there are more specialized tests such as defecography or anorectal manometry that should be performed first to better determine what the problem is and if there is an alternative non-operative treatment that could work, such as biofeedback to train the pelvic floor muscles to help you evacuate properly.

2. A patient with refractory gastroesophageal reflux disease (GERD).

    (a) Similar to the first example, perhaps what you really have is not even GERD. Sometimes what patients have is dyspepsia, bile duct stones, or a pancreatic disorder that is mistaken as GERD. If it is not burning under your chest and/or you do not feel liquid or food coming back up from your stomach, there is a very good chance that what you have is not GERD.

(b) Also similar to the first example, the GERD medication you have tried may not have been the right one or at the right dose, or maybe you did not give it enough time to take effect. In addition, perhaps you were not taking it properly. For instance, GERD medications belonging to the proton pump inhibitor (PPI) class, such as omeprazole, pantoprazole, and lansoprazole, should be taken approximately 30 min *before* a meal; I have seen many patients who were taking these medications *after* meals, and upon uncovering this and modifying the timing of the medications, experienced GERD symptom relief.

(c) GERD tends to be a long-term problem, so if you come off the medication once your symptoms have resolved, it is quite likely that they will come back in a matter of weeks or months, sometimes even sooner. This does not mean the treatment failed or that there is something seriously wrong, but not every patient or provider knows this. The same can be said about example 1 (constipation) as well.

(d) You may be doing things that cause GERD that can be modified, e.g. laying down right after eating or eating acidic foods (marinara sauce, vinegar, citrus) or large fatty meals.

(e) Lastly, some patients are referred for anti-GERD surgery; realize that these are typically major undertakings that don't always go as planned (i.e. complications may arise), that there may be less invasive options, and that even if all goes well, you may still need to stay on anti-acid medication afterward.

3. A patient with problematic "hemorrhoids".

(a) Unbeknownst to many, hemorrhoids are structures that we all have, albeit to varying degrees, from small and unnoticeable to large and bothersome. Hemorrhoids are veins around the anus that tend to become enlarged with prolonged straining or sitting due to pooling of blood in them. This knowledge helps dispel myths and alleviate worries.

(b) There are actually two main types of hemorrhoids: internal and external. Internal and external hemorrhoids, although in close proximity, are quite different—they cause different symptoms and are treated differently—yet tend to be lumped together and a cause of confusion. In a nutshell, I will say internal hemorrhoids can bleed whereas external hemorrhoids can itch or hurt.

(c) Although many people are bothered by hemorrhoids (internal or external), it is important to not assume that your problem is just hemorrhoids. There are other conditions which can masquerade as hemorrhoids; I have seen patients think that they have hemorrhoids whereas in fact they have rectal cancer, inflammatory bowel disease, or rectal prolapse (three very different diagnoses!). If you think you have hemorrhoids, it is usually ok to empirically treat for such for a brief period of time and assess the response; if the problem (bleeding or pain or otherwise) persists despite treatment, that is a sign that you need further evaluation to make sure you do not have some other, more serious problem. Most primary care providers cannot complete the necessary evaluation, thus a referral to a specialist is indicated.

(d) While internal hemorrhoids can be categorized as a problem under the umbrella of gastroenterology (GI), there are many gastroenterologists who do not perform hemorrhoidal treatment procedures, and sometimes internal hemorrhoids are too big for a gastroenterologist to treat and instead require surgical intervention. If you are suffering with hemorrhoids and your provider is not able to help you, you need not settle; a second opinion, such as from a colorectal surgeon, may illuminate additional treatment options.

A second opinion can come in handy at a variety of ways and junctures in each of the three aforementioned cases. Some patients will suffer for years before seeking out a second opinion, whereas others will obtain one early on. If in doubt, bring up the subject with your confidants and see what advice you may be given (Fig. 11.1).

Putting it all Together

A second opinion can help you gain the perspective of more than one reasonable mind and potentially uncover possibilities and options that have not been entertained or pursued. There are many scenarios in which a second opinion can be helpful and many benefits a second opinion can provide, though the process can seem somewhat nebulous or daunting. An individualized approach is important to decide if and when to obtain a second opinion, and there are various ways to best go about it. For those who have an inkling that a second opinion would be helpful, my experience has been that more often than not, it is.

This chapter concludes Part 3 of this book. Next, in Part 4, we will explore treatments and solutions for digestive problems, recognizing that each patient is unique, and one size does not fit all. Starting with Chap. 12, we will cover initial approaches, in particular lifestyle and dietary modifications.

Further Reading

Can a second opinion make a difference? News. Yale Medicine.
Extent of diagnostic agreement among medical referrals. PubMed (nih.gov).
FAQs about rare diseases. Genetic and Rare Diseases Information Center (GARD)—an NCATS Program (nih.gov).
Need a second opinion? Here's what to say to your doctor (webmd.com).
When and how to get a second opinion. Winchester Hospital.
Why you should consider a second medical opinion. Cleveland Clinic.

Part IV
Treatments and Solutions: Each Patient Is Unique, and One Size Doesn't Fit All

Chapter 12
Initial Approaches: Lifestyle and Dietary Modifications

The Association Between Lifestyle, Diet, and Digestive Problems

Eastern (e.g. Chinese) and other forms of traditional medicine have long recognized the close relationship between one's lifestyle and diet and one's health and longevity. Modern medicine has similarly found that the development of many digestive problems is closely associated with factors such as exercise, sleep, work, consumption of alcohol and tobacco, and diet, among others (Fig. 12.1). These factors are also therefore associated with the treatment and course of digestive problems. Thus, it is important to comprehensively explore lifestyle and dietary factors when evaluating digestive problems and recognize that they can be modified for therapeutic benefit.

For better or worse, not every digestive problem has a strong association with lifestyle and dietary factors. There are some scenarios where you may modify your lifestyle or diet, but your digestive problem may not budge, although you may reap other benefits, such as cardiovascular. There are also scenarios where your digestive problem may improve, but you might need an additional intervention as well, like a medication, to adequately treat the problem. Interestingly, some of the aforementioned associations are fairly common-sense, whereas others are subtle or unexpected; involvement of a healthcare provider is often needed to uncover the latter.

J. H. Tabibian, *Digestive Problems Solved*, https://doi.org/10.1007/978-3-031-16317-3_12

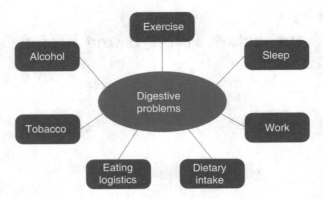

Fig. 12.1 Lifestyle and dietary factors which may contribute to various digestive problems and potentially be modified for therapeutic purposes.
Legend: Shown here are various lifestyle and dietary factors which may contribute to digestive problems and can be considered as potential areas to modify for the purpose of achieving therapeutic benefit. These factors can evolve over time with the aging process. Note that this list is not exhaustive given there are other factors (aside from lifestyle and dietary), as discussed in other chapters, which may contribute to digestive problems

Areas for Reflection and Potential Modification

It may be difficult to know where to begin with lifestyle and dietary modifications. Certain modifications may make obvious sense for your digestive problem, whereas others may not. Overall, functional gastrointestinal (GI) disorders are most likely to benefit from lifestyle and dietary modifications, but there is certainly potential for improvement or even prevention with various organic GI disorders as well. Admittedly, some thoughtful trial-and-error may be needed to find what lifestyle and dietary modifications are the best fit for your scenario. Many times, there's room for more than one modification, though it is typically best to go one at a time.

In no particular order, below are some lifestyle and dietary areas that you could reflect on, asking yourself "might this be playing a role with my digestive problem?", and potentially modify with the hopes of deriving therapeutic benefit. As you reflect on the these, keep in mind that there are some changes that you might be able to make on your own, whereas others would be best embarked upon in conjunction with your healthcare provider or some other professional, such as a registered dietician or physical therapist. When in doubt, err toward seeking the input of a healthcare professional; they may shed additional light on the matter and help make modifications more effective.

Exercise

Exercise has so many benefits—and it is not just about losing weight or becoming toned. Exercise has been found to protect against various digestive problems, such as nonalcoholic fatty liver disease, diverticular disease, and even esophageal cancer, to name just a few. In addition, it can help de-stress your mind, which can help your body carry out regular GI activities such as a normal appetite or effective bowel movement, in addition to helping you cope with the challenges life may throw at you. We do not fully understand all of the GI benefits of exercise, but as with the non-GI benefits, there are seemingly many. For example, I have seen plenty of patients who experience less gastroesophageal reflux and/or less bloating when they engage in regular exercise, and even more so when exercise leads to loss of excess weight. If exercise is not your thing because you are not aiming to be buff or have an ultra-toned body, recognize that there are plenty other benefits that can be derived. If you are on the fence, I would say exercise is worth a try, whether it is getting on a treadmill, elliptical, stationary bike, going out for a brisk stroll, or one of many other forms; you might just be surprised for the better.

Sleep

Sleep and digestive problems have numerous interrelated associations. Based on research to date, these changes are likely related, at least in part, to disruption of the circadian rhythm, or our "internal clock". For example, patients with gastroesophageal reflux as well as those with irritable bowel syndrome (IBS) often report sleep disorders/poor sleep quality, such as nocturnal awakening or morning fatigue. Additionally, sleep disorders can induce and aggravate the symptoms of IBS, and poor sleep quality decreases the threshold of visceral (or GI) pain, thus making it more apparent. Indeed, sleep disorders have been associated with the severity of symptoms and the comorbidity of anxiety in patients with functional GI disorders, including but not limited to IBS. Moreover, inadequate or disrupted sleep can lead to irregular bowel habits, especially a tendency toward constipation. Suffice it to say, if you have sleep issues and also a digestive problem, there is a good chance the two could be interrelated and that addressing the former could lead to improvement in the latter (Fig. 12.1).

Work Dynamics

Work, and by extension school, are important in the context of digestive problems for at least a few reasons. First, certain digestive problems, for example IBS, are more common in those working rotating shifts or night shifts compared to those working only day shifts. Much of this is probably related to issues with sleep quality and circadian rhythm disruption, but there may be other factors too, such as the social isolation of a night shift, the hassle of rotating shifts, and so forth. Second, work stress can wear us down and cause or aggravate digestive problems, be they heartburn, nausea, abdominal pain, appetite loss, or bowel habit changes. I would be lying if I said work or school stressors have never had a negative impact on my GI system or led me to transiently experience digestive problems, especially nausea and loss of appetite; this actually was an impetus for me conducting a study on resident physician wellbeing while I was in training (see Further Reading section for reference). Third, work may expose us to activities such as heavy lifting, non-ergonomic body positions, and inhaling fumes, which can predispose us to or worsen certain digestive problems; a common example would be hemorrhoids worsened by prolonged seating, as may be the case with a secretary or truck driver, or by heavy lifting. Fourth, a grueling work schedule may prevent us from addressing our physiological needs, such as eating on time or going to the restroom when we have an urge to have a bowel movement, and can thus cause or worsen digestive problems. Overall, once you recognize the link between your work dynamics and your digestive problems, this can open up various options that you might pursue to try to make things better.

Drinking and Smoking

There are abundant published data indicating an association between both alcohol and/or tobacco consumption and various digestive problems. Some of these associations are fairly well known, whereas others are not and may thus be quite surprising to patients. To name a few associations:

- Alcohol is a solvent and can thus cause direct irritation to the lining of the digestive tract, especially the esophagus and stomach. It can also alter gastric acid secretion and predispose to gastroesophageal acid reflux, causing irritation and potential ulceration in the esophagus and/or stomach. These effects are amplified by the amount of alcohol taken in, but even small amounts of alcohol can cause clinically-evident problems in some individuals. For example, some people with existing acid reflux can notice significant worsening with a half glass or less of red wine. Alcohol can also cause inflammation of the pancreas due to both binge drinking, which can cause acute pancreatitis, and long-term drinking, which can cause chronic pancreatitis. Thus, the well known association between long-term excess alcohol intake and liver disease is just one aspect of how alcohol is associated with digestive problems.
- Smoking tobacco has been associated with various digestive problems under the umbrella of "dyspepsia," which in lay terms is also referred to as "gastritis" or "indigestion". These may include symptoms of early fullness, upper abdominal pain, heartburn, or nausea. Smoking can also decrease the production of saliva, which impairs the ability of the esophagus to cope with acid exposure, whether it is acid from what we eat or reflux from the stomach. It can also lead to increased

production of gastric acid, thus aggravating the matter futher. Similar to alcohol, smoking can also cause worsening of *existing* digestive problems, such as gastro-esophageal reflux and Crohn's disease, an inflammatory disorder of the GI system. Though lung cancer tends to be the malignancy that comes to mind when thinking about smoking, there is also an association with cancers of the esophagus, colon, and pancreas, among others. If an individual who smokes also drinks alcohol, this can pose a double blow to the GI system.

I'm often asked if I recommend complete abstinence from alcohol, and despite the aforementioned hazards, I actually seldom say yes. Alcohol can provide some health benefits, which I do not discount. Nevertheless, I generally suggest focusing on quality rather than quantity, such as having a little bit of a beverage you really like. There are cases, though, where even a small amount of alcohol can be harmful, so every case is different. With regard to smoking, I never encourage a patient to keep smoking, but I also realize how difficult it can be to quit, and that it is easier said than done. But once over the hump of quitting, I cannot recall a single person who has not said that they are feeling better overall and/or in regard to their digestive problems. It is worthwhile to at least consult with your healthcare provider and ask if alcohol or smoking could be related to your problems. If so, you may have some important changes to implement.

Dietary Intake

It should be no surprise that when it comes to digestive problems, what you eat can be an important factor. Certain foods are closely associated with certain digestive problems, and notably, even "healthy" foods can cause digestive problems in certain individuals. For example:

- Citrus, onions, marinara sauce, vinegar, coffee, and red wine can all cause or worsen heartburn and/or gastroesophageal reflux.
- Milk and other lactose-containing dairy products, beans, and carbonated drinks often result in gas/ bloating.
- Gluten-containing foods are the trigger of small intestinal inflammation in those with Celiac disease, but even individuals who do not have Celiac disease can be sensitive to gluten-containing foods and develop symptoms such as bloating and nausea from them.
- Fatty foods can cause a sensation of heaviness, predispose one to gastroesophageal reflux, and/or trigger an urgent bowel movement, known as the "gastrocolic reflex".
- Some foods, such as spinach, breads, and potatoes, tend to be constipating. Others, including sugary foods, caffeinated beverages, and artificial sweeteners, tend to lead to looser stools. Depending on one's bowel habits, this can make matters better or worse.

The list goes on and on and can apply to many different digestive problems, including dyspepsia, IBS, nonalcoholic fatty liver disease, and diverticular disease. Interestingly, even the temperature of your food can be associated with digestive problems; one sobering example is that very hot food and beverage, if consumed repeatedly over years, can predispose to esophageal cancer. Therefore, if you have a digestive problem, there is a good chance that you are eating something that is making it worse or that there is something you can modify in your diet that can make it better. It might be a matter of cutting out lactose, avoiding acidic substances, eating more fiber, having less fatty meals, or something else. It largely depends on what your particular digestive problem is and what your baseline diet consists of, and awareness is key. I suggest a consultation with a registered dietitian for many patients to help them pay closer attention to their body and digestive problems and identify dietary areas wherein therapeutic modifications can be made.

Specific Diets

While making small modifications to dietary intake is effective for some individuals, others will need or want a dietary overhaul per se. There are various specific diets out there, some of which can be useful for those with digestive problems. As there are entire books written just on the topic of diets, I will only briefly mention two:

- The first is the low FODMAP diet, which is a diet low in the components of the acronym "FODMAP": fermentable oligosaccharides, disaccharides, monosaccharides, and polyols (Table 12.1). These components, when ingested and acted upon by intestinal bacteria, cause the production and release of gas. I find this diet to be highly useful for those with IBS, small intestinal bacterial overgrowth, bloating, and/or excess belching or flatulence, and there are numerous studies out there to support it.
- The second is the specific carbohydrate diet, which has shown benefit in not only functional but also organic GI disorders, such as inflammatory bowel disease. This diet tends to be quite restrictive, permitting only foods which are unprocessed and free of grain and certain sugars and starches. I know some patients who have tried a modified, slightly less strict version of this diet, and it has helped with their digestive problems.

A couple other diets that have merit are the Mediterranean diet and the Paleo, or "caveman", diet. A number of these diets have overlapping features, and I think any of them could be beneficial for a given person, depending on the circumstance. At the very least, diet is often a topic worth reviewing with your healthcare provider and/or dietician in the context of your particular digestive problem and overall health needs. Notably, as many will know, a gluten-free diet is the mainstay of

Table 12.1 Foods groups and FODMAP content of their constituents

Food group/ category	Low FODMAP content	High FODMAP content
Vegetables and legumes	Alfalfa, bean sprouts, butternut squash, carrots, celery, chick peas, chives, collard greens, corn, cucumber, eggplant, green beans, ginger, lentils, lettuce, soy/tofu, tomatoes	Artichoke, asparagus, beans (e.g. kidney, black), Brussels sprouts, cassava, cauliflower, garlic, okra, onion, mange tout, mushrooms, peas, savoy cabbage
Fruit	Bananas, blueberries, cantaloupe, cranberry, citrus (e.g. mandarin, orange), grapes, kiwi, passion fruit, papaya, pineapple, raspberry, strawberry, tamarind	Apples, apricots, avocado, blackberries, currants, cherries, dates, goji berries, grapefruit, lychee, mango, nectarines, peaches, pears, persimmon, pineapple, plums, watermelon
Meats and seafood	Beef, chicken, lamb, pork, turkey, fish (e.g., cod, salmon, trout, tuna), seafood (e.g., crab, lobster, mussels, oysters, shrimp)	Chorizo, salami, sausage, other processed meats
Cereals, grains, and nuts	Bulgur, buckwheat, chestnuts, cornflour, macadamia nuts, peanuts, pecans, pine nuts, polenta, popcorn, potato flour, quinoa, rice, walnuts	Almonds, amaranth flour, barley, bran/oats, bread (unless wheat- and gluten-free), cashews, cous cous, gnocchi, pistachios, rye, semolina, spelt flour
Dairy	Butter, eggs, hard (fermented) cheese, margarine, whipped cream	Milk, buttermilk, soft or fresh cheese, sour cream, ice cream, custard, gelato, kefir
Sweets and condiments	Aspartame, capers, malted chocolate, olive oil, soy sauce, stevia, sucralose, table sugar, vinegars	Agave, fructose, hummus, honey, pesto sauce, relish/vegetable pickle, sorbitol, tahini paste, xylitol

Legend: When following a low FODMAP diet, foods that are have high FODMAP content should be avoided, as these will typically tend to cause more gas and bloating. In some individuals, some such foods can be gradually re-introduced one-by-one (i.e. don't add multiple high FODMAP foods back into your diet at once), as tolerated. Conversely, some low FODMAP foods, for whatever reason, may not be tolerated by certain individuals (e.g. due to miscellaneous food sensitivities) and thus should be avoided. It's often best to let your body decide.
Note: (1) many high FODMAP dairy products will have lactose-free varieties which can be considered low FODMAP, (2) this list is not exhaustive, and (3) some foods (e.g. whipped cream) may be considered high FODMAP if greater than a normal serving size is consumed.

treatment for those with Celiac disease, though it can also be helpful in those who have non-Celiac gluten intolerance, as can a low-FODMAP diet.

With essentially any diet you end up choosing, some trial and error is permissible, if not necessary. A diet need not be set in stone, and it can be fine-tuned based on how it works for you and your digestive problem and health goals. For instance, even though yogurt is listed as a high FODMAP food, many patients will attest that it makes them feel better, with less bloating, pain, and nausea. So you have to listen to your body. Flexibility and attentive monitoring are important. Personally, I tend to follow a mix between a Mediterranean diet and a Paleo diet for general as well as GI health.

Eating Logistics

Going hand-in-hand with what you eat are your eating logistics, or how you eat and your habits around mealtime. Eating logistics can have an important association with various digestive problems, especially those involving the upper digestive tract. There are some relatively simple and safe interventions in this regard that can be tried to see if they bring you some relief, such as the following:

- Eat smaller and more frequent meals rather than a few large meals. This can help mitigate bloating, reflux, and too strong of a gastrocolic reflux, which can produce a sudden urge to have a bowel movement (known as "fecal urgency"), among other benefits.
- Take your time eating and refrain from gulping down your food or drink. This can help avoid an excess intake of calories, inadvertent swallowing of air and associated belching and bloating, and also too strong of a gastrocolic reflex.
- Try not to lie down for at least two, and preferably three, hours after a meal. This can decrease reflux and heartburn since gravity can help keep gastric acid and other contents down rather than refluxing back up into the esophagus (an effect that is lost when you lie down too soon).
- Avoid fatty and acidic foods, especially at night or anytime you think you may lie down relatively soon after eating. This can help decrease reflux and heartburn.

These are just a few potential interventions and benefits. The list is not exhaustive, but it highlights how there is more to eating than just what you eat. I've come across many patients who have experienced considerable improvement in their digestive problems just with modification of their eating logistics.

Changes that Come with the Aging Process

Aging is a dynamic, multifaceted process during which our bodies undergo myriad changes. Our lifestyle and dietary habits tend to also change as we age. Moreover, our body's ability to cope with our lifestyle and dietary habits may become diminished as we age. I, for one, am not as active and do not eat the same foods or the same way as when I was in my teens. The biological, physiological, and other changes that come along with the aging process can have far-reaching and intertwined impact. I would be remiss were I to not mention aging in this chapter and provide a few real-world examples as they relate to digestive problems.

Lactose Intolerance and Food Sensitivity

Millions of people across the world are intolerant to lactose, a sugar found in dairy products, because they are born lacking "lactase," the intestinal enzyme that breaks down lactose. Upon consumption of lactose, individuals with lactose intolerance will experience symptoms such as abdominal cramps, bloating, flatus, and/or diarrhea. In addition to those who are born lactose intolerant, many individuals will *become* lactose intolerant later in life due to decreased intestinal production of lactase. This is often a gradual change, but sometimes it can be or seem quick in onset. One common scenario is when someone becomes lactose intolerant following a GI infection, as the perturbed small intestine stops producing sufficient lactase. Lactose intolerance can sound trivial, but it is an official diagnosis that can be quite bothersome, though generally not dangerous per se. Therefore, a low hanging fruit in someone with symptoms of lactose intolerance is to consider a trial of a lactose-free diet or to take a lactase supplement anytime lactose-containing foods are consumed. Many patients will notice improvement quite quickly—within a day or two—if lactose intolerance is the underlying cause of their digestive problems.

Somewhat akin to lactose intolerance, over time we may develop a sensitivity to certain foods such that we cannot eat them the way we used to. The reasons for this are not as clear-cut as not having enough of the right digestive enzyme and instead are probably multifactorial. To provide a personal example, I cannot eat garlic or drink red wine the way I used to in my 20s; garlic now causes me to feel full, bloated, and belch, whereas red wine (depending on the specific type) leads me to have heartburn the next morning. Given the lack of "red flags" (Chap. 3) in my case, rather than going and having scans and other tests performed, I just choose to avoid garlic and red wine or prepare myself for the side effects I'll be feeling. It is important to make a note of foods that do not sit well with us and listen to our bodies. If you notice a dietary intolerance or sensitivity, see if avoiding the food or beverage alleviates your digestive problem. When in doubt, discuss with your healthcare provider to be on the safe side.

A Tendency Toward Constipation

As we become older, our GI system tends to slow down, predisposing us to constipation. There are various reasons for this slow down, both known and unknown. Two important considerations that intersect with aging in this context are sleep and exercise. We tend to need less sleep both as we get older and as our physical activity decreases, and the amount we sleep affects the function of our GI system as discussed earlier. Indeed, research has shown that both decreased and increased sleep are correlated with constipation. The way I see it, if you undersleep, you have not given your body the opportunity to rest sufficiently to prepare for a bowel movement; if you oversleep, your body is interpreting it as a sign to slow things down. In a nutshell, sleep disturbance can lead to bowel disturbance. With this in mind, I believe it is important to ask our older patients about sleep because of the particular impact it can have on their GI system.

Exercise is also useful for maintaining bowel regularity in older adults. We often need a little extra oomph to stay regular as we age, and exercise can fit this bill, helping to whip our GI system into shape. Many older individuals cannot or do not exercise, and instead become sedentary. As a result, they may become reliant on stool softeners to achieve regularity. It is ok to use stool softeners, but if I could pick between exercise vs. pills for a given patient to stay regular, my preference would be the former. Some people will need more than just one form of extra oomph, such as exercise and a stool softener, and of course you shouldn't forget the role of diet. Ironically, I know of some people who have become both lactose intolerant and constipated over the years and leveraged the former to manage the latter; that is, they intentionally consume dairy products as a natural remedy for their constipation. This approach may of course produce the side effects of bloating and flatus, but for some these are preferable over having to take stool softeners.

Diverticulosis and Diverticular Disease

Diverticulosis refers to the formation or presence of "diverticula," or little outpouchings in the wall of a hollow structure. In the GI system, diverticulosis becomes more prevalent with age and most often occurs in the colon, though it can also form in the small intestine, gallbladder, or other organs. In most individuals, diverticulosis of the colon does not lead to problems. In some individuals, however, a diverticulum can become inflamed or bleed, which are the two main manifestations of diverticular disease. The cause of diverticulosis, and for that matter diverticular disease, is not precisely understood. Aside from age, one risk factor seems to be constipation, while protection seems to be conferred by certain lifestyle and dietary factors, such as exercise, fiber intake, and avoidance of saturated fat and red meat. What this means is that in order to avoid developing diverticulosis or diverticular disease, you may need to make certain modifications, such as increasing exercise, increasing fiber intake from vegetables, grains, or over-the-counter supplements, and decreasing saturated fat and red meat intake. These modifications also happen to be protective against colorectal cancer, so think of this as a nice fringe benefit.

There is a lingering misconception that those who have diverticulosis must avoid nuts and seeds, the thought being that they become stuck inside diverticula. Though this notion has been debunked in the medical literature, there still are patients who tell me that whenever they eat popcorn or strawberries, their diverticulosis flares up. I am not exactly sure how to explain this, but I do not argue with it—I just tell them that despite what current literature says for patients in general, they might as well listen to their body and not eat the foods that seem to cause them bothersome symptoms. On the other hand, if you have diverticulosis and love eating popcorn, strawberries, nuts, or seeds and feel fine when you do, you may carry on.

Putting it all Together

It has been long recognized that how we live and what we eat are interrelated with our health and how we feel. By extension, our lifestyle and diet are closely related with whether or not we develop digestive problems. Though implementing lifestyle and dietary modifications is not always easy—after all, some habits are hard to break—doing so is generally safe, free, and in many instances quite effective. In this chapter, we reviewed lifestyle and dietary modifications as initial approaches to managing digestive problems. What exactly should be modified, whether it's exercise, sleep, alcohol intake, diet, eating logistics, or something else, will depend on the individual and the specific digestive problem. Certain modifications will make more sense and be more effective in certain scenarios. Sometimes it is obvious what needs to be modified, but other times the connection is less clear, and a healthcare provider may be needed to provide input and guidance. Some digestive problems are just part of the aging process, but even these can often be alleviated through lifestyle and dietary modifications. At times, these modifications are helpful but not quite enough to fully manage a digestive problem, and thus a combination approach may be needed. Next, in Chap. 13, we discuss over-the-counter and prescription medications for treatment of digestive problems.

Further Reading

Alcoholic disease: liver and beyond. PubMed (nih.gov).
Behavioral gastroenterology: an emerging system and new frontier of action. PubMed (nih.gov).
Decreased sleep associated with constipation among U.S adults (healio.com).
Diet & lifestyle changes. About GERD.
Dietary fiber and the risk of acute diverticulitis. PubMed (nih.gov).
Disturbed sleep and disturbed bowel functions: implications for constipation in healthy individuals. PubMed (nih.gov).
https://pubmed.ncbi.nlm.nih.gov/31897450/
Lifestyle changes. About Kids GI.
Lifestyle changes for gastroesophageal reflux disease. NYU Langone Health.
Sleep disturbances are linked to both upper and lower gastrointestinal symptoms in the general population. PubMed (nih.gov).
Smoking status and prevalence of upper gastrointestinal disorders. PubMed (nih.gov).

Chapter 13
Over-the-Counter and Prescription Medications

OTC Medications for Digestive Disorders

The OTC medication market is massive, but there is a small handful of OTC medications which constitute the majority of what is taken for digestive problems. An overview of these medications is provided in Table 13.1.

Advantages of OTC Medications

From a healthcare provider's perspective, there are a couple reasons why it is good that OTC medications exist. Just as there is a progressive sequence in diagnostic testing from less to more invasive, as covered in Chap. 9, there is often a progressive sequence in treatment from less to more risky or from less to more costly. OTC medications can be regarded as a relatively early step in the sequence, and not everyone with digestive problems will need to progress to prescription medications. It is also nice that patients have options readily available to them to trial and error in pursuit of relief, at least when their digestive problems are mild and in the absence of red flags (Chap. 3), rather than necessitating a medical appointment.

From a patient's perspective, OTC medications can have many advantages, including:

- Quick and on demand; you might in fact already have some in your home. For many OTC medications, you can take them essentially whenever you feel. Of course, caution is necessary to not exceed the dose indicated on the label.
- Widely accessible. OTC medications are usually available at pharmacies, supermarkets, and even gas stations. You have flexible choices in this regard.

J. H. Tabibian, *Digestive Problems Solved*, https://doi.org/10.1007/978-3-031-16317-3_13

Table 13.1 Overview of commonly used over-the-counter medications for digestive problems

Medication	How it works	What it's used for	Things to bear in mind
Antacids (e.g. tums, Mylanta, and generics)	Neutralize acid in the upper digestive tract	Relief of heartburn, acid indigestion	• These medicines simply neutralize the acid present and don't prevent more from being form. • Relatively weak but can be useful for infrequent and mild acid-related symptoms. • There can be drug-drug interactions. • Caution in those with kidney impairment.
Bismuth subsalicylate (e.g. PeptoBismol® and generics)	Anti-secretory and anti-inflammatory effects	Relief of dyspepsia (including acid indigestion, nausea, bloating) and of diarrhea	• Can help ease a variety of digestive problems. • There can be drug-drug interactions. • Constipation can occur. • Stools may turn dark/black.
Docusate (e.g. Colace® and generics)	Reduces surface tension of the oil-water interface of the stool resulting in enhanced incorporation of water into stool	Relief of constipation (to soften stool)	• Very safe when used at recommended doses. • Relatively weak medication but can be useful for mild constipation or in conjunction with other approaches. • Not a stimulant laxative, thus should not expect it to "make you go"
Fiber supplements (e.g. Metamucil®, Citrucel®, Benefiber®, and generics)	Soluble fiber absorbs water in the intestine to form a viscous liquid and provide a soft bulking effect	Relief of constipation or diarrhea. Prevent complications of diverticulosis	• Can serve as an "averaging" agent (i.e. helpful with people with stools that are too soft/watery or too hard). • Not all fiber is the same; psyllium fiber (as opposed to methycellulose or wheat dextrin) tends to cause bloating. • Should not use if any concern of possible gastrointestinal narrowing/blockage.

Table 13.1 (continued)

Medication	How it works	What it's used for	Things to bear in mind
Histamine-2 receptor blockers (e.g. Zantac, Pepcid, and generics)	Blocks histamine from binding to receptors on gastric parietal cells, thus inhibiting acid secretion	Relief of gastroesophageal reflux disease	• Stronger than antacids, though over time can lose efficacy; not as strong as proton pump inhibitor (PPI) medications. • There can be drug-drug interactions. • Caution in those with kidney impairment.
Loperamide (e.g. Imodium® and generics)	Blocks intestinal muscle contractions, decreases secretions	Relief of diarrhea	• Generally safe when used at recommended doses. • Can quickly overshoot to constipation
Polyethylene glycol (e.g. MiraLAX® and generics)	Causes water retention (through a process called osmosis) in the stool	Relief of constipation (to soften stool)	• Very safe when used at recommended doses. • Not a stimulant laxative, thus should not expect it to "make you go". • Using too much may cause diarrhea.
Simethicone (gas-X® and generics)	Decreases the surface tension of gas bubbles thereby disperses and prevents gas pockets in the GI system	Relief of bloating	• Very safe when used at recommended doses. • Can provide short-term relief of bloating. • May need dietary or other modifications to best manage bloating.

Provided herein is a high-level view of common indications; information is not exhaustive. Remember also that prolonged symptoms should generally prompt an evaluation by a healthcare provider.

- Doesn't require going through insurance; you can go and buy them without having to wait for insurance approval. Avoiding the hassle of insurance is a nice feature, though some OTC medications can be pricey without insurance coverage.
- Many options. Often times there is more than one brand of an OTC medication. There may also be different formulations, such as a pill, powder, or liquid. In addition, there may be multiple OTC medications for a given digestive disorder, like for heartburn (for instance, antacids, histamine-2 receptor blockers, and proton pump inhibitors).
- Generally safe. Most OTC medications are safe in the sense that when the directions on the label are followed, you typically do not have to worry about adverse side effects (though allergic reactions can potentially occur), at least not to the

same extent as with prescription medications. There are some exceptions, however, so you should make sure to read the package and consider discussing with the pharmacist and/or your healthcare provider prior to use.

- Empowering. Having OTC medication options gives you the power and capacity to try to take control of your digestive problem, and many times you are able to without needing to go further down the diagnostic or treatment sequence.

Disadvantages to OTC Medications

Though it is difficult to deny the major role that OTC medications have in the management of digestive problems, there are also some important drawbacks to recognize. With so many different digestive problems and so many different OTC medications, things do not always go favorably in every case. Some fundamental drawbacks of OTC medication use include the possibility that it may be:

- Acting as a bandaid rather than a true treatment. Imagine a patient who has diarrhea due to inflammatory bowel disease (IBD). It is different than diarrhea due to irritable bowel syndrome, microscopic colitis, or infection. Thus, it needs to be treated accordingly, with something that addresses the intestinal inflammation and injury inherent to IBD. Therefore, even if an OTC anti-diarrheal medication stops the diarrhea, it could just be covering up the underlying issue rather than preventing damage to the bowels, as may be achieved with the appropriate medications for treatment of IBD, such as anti-inflammatories and immunosuppressants.
- Unwittingly trying to treat the wrong digestive problem and/or delaying accurate diagnosis. A grim example of this would be pain in the upper abdomen that is thought to be due to "gastritis". It would be ok to empirically try acid suppression medications, and if they result in resolution of symptoms, great; but if not, an evaluation by a healthcare provider is needed rather than spending time continuing the same medication and hoping that it will eventually work. After all, the pain could be coming from the pancreas or some other structure for which acid suppression is not the right treatment. Another example would be rectal bleeding. If it is occurring in the setting of constipation and straining, it is probably benign and due to irritation of internal hemorrhoids, and hence it would be reasonable to take OTC stool softeners; but if the bleeding is not resolving after a couple weeks, or if it is arising in the absence of a plausible benign explanation, this would point to a need for an evaluation by a healthcare provider. These could be signs of colorectal cancer, and thus stool softeners alone would be misguided.
- Undertreating the correct problem. Let us imagine you experience heartburn. You start an OTC medication and are content with the response you are having to it, though you may still have some breakthrough heartburn periodically. Despite feeling better, it is possible there is still acid exposure to the esophagus,

which can predispose to various complications over time, including Barrett's esophagus, esophageal strictures, and even esophageal cancer. Therefore, it may be that you need more treatment, such as the prescription strength version of the medication, the prescription strength medication coupled with lifestyle changes (Chap. 12), or some other approach other than just the OTC medication. If you were to just stay on the OTC medication and not consult with a healthcare provider about your problem, the problem could fester in the background and result in esophageal injury and complications over time. Indeed, for many digestive problems, there is a discord between symptomatic control and clinical control; sometimes you may feel fine, but when evaluated more closely with blood tests, a scan, or endoscopy, there is objective evidence of an undertreated problem.

- A cause of untoward effects. Though generally safe, especially at the doses recommended on the medication label, some OTC medications can and do have adverse side effects. Just because a medication is OTC does not mean it is safe or right for you.
- Available instead by prescription. Some OTC medications may be prescribed, depending on the specific medication, dose, and/or insurance plan. Having these medications prescribed can have a couple benefits over buying them as OTC. First, it may make the medication less costly, as the copayment may be less than the OTC price. Second, it provides extra reassurance knowing that the recommendation to use the medication is coming from a healthcare provider.

Overall, I would say that if you are going to try OTC medications, at least speak to the pharmacist where you are shopping for some advice on which medication is most suitable for you. You may receive useful input, be steered away from potential pitfalls, and maybe even be advised to see a healthcare provider on the basis of what the pharmacist makes of your digestive problem. If in doubt, it is certainly reasonable to speak with your healthcare provider from the outset before deciding to try an OTC medication.

Prescription Medications for Digestive Problems: Guiding Principles

Many digestive problems will ultimately require treatment with a prescription medication. Whether or not a prescription medication is required, and its dosage and duration, will depend on the nature and severity of the digestive problem and the healthcare professional's assessment. For instance, treatment of *H. pylori* infection in the stomach generally consists of a few prescription medications, but only for 10–14 days. On the other hand, gastroesophageal reflux disease (GERD) may require a prescription acid suppression medicine for life. As these medications are, by definition, being taken by the recommendation of a qualified and licensed healthcare professional, you should already have a good resource on hand (the prescriber). Therefore, I will be brief here and focus on some important principles that you should bear in mind as an informed patient and self-advocate. Most of these principles are applicable not only to prescription medications, but also OTC medications.

Starting Dose

For many if not most medications, there is a range of doses at which treatment can be initiated. In the absence of a single starting dose, the question may arise as to how high of a dose to start with. The concern with starting low is that it may not be sufficient, which can lead to two issues: the premature perception that the medication is not helping as well as the problem persisting until the dose is sufficiently increased. The concern with starting high is that it may not be tolerated well and that you may develop an adverse effect. In general, the best choice for a starting dose depends on the particular digestive problem, your priorities, and input from your healthcare provider. For those with GERD or similar acid-related problems, we will often start at a medium- or high-dose of acid suppression medication, such as a PPI. Examples of a PPI medication include esomeprazole, under the brand Nexium® or the "purple pill", or pantoprazole, under the brand name Protonix®. One reason for doing so is that PPI medication is very safe, especially short-term. Another is that if there is no response to a high dose, you can move on to something else relatively soon, as opposed to trying a low-dose and then trying a higher dose for several more weeks to months. But this practice is not universal, and some providers, especially in primary care, may prefer to start low with a step-up approach.

How to Take

How a medication should be taken is a sizable topic and one wherein detail can be quite important. It encompasses how often to take it, when to take it in respect to food, taking it in the morning vs. at night, and so forth and is important to optimize outcomes, in particular to maximize benefit and minimize adverse effects. Continuing with the example of acid suppression medication such as a PPI, it is best to take 30–45 minutes before mealtime to achieve maximum benefit. Many patients are not told or do not know this, but making this simple change can result in symptom resolution when the medication is otherwise apparently not working. There are also times where a medication is prescribed to be taken two, three, or four times a day, but in reality, it can be taken all at the same time for simplicity's sake. It is worth asking about, as multiple times a day dosing can be burdensome and difficult to adhere to, though sometimes it is in fact necessary depending on the medication.

When to Anticipate the Medication to Take Effect

There is often a misconception that if a medication is prescribed it is going to work immediately. It is possible that it will start to work immediately, but that does not necessarily mean you will notice improvement immediately; indeed, it might take days to weeks for the effect of the medication to become noticeable. This is the case with a number of medications used to treat digestive problems, such as PPIs and stool softeners, among others. Unfortunately, as with starting with too low a dose, this misconception of immediate improvement can be a cause for premature discontinuation of a medication and concluding that "it did not work for me," which is not an uncommon occurrence. It is important for healthcare providers to discuss and for patients to ask about when to expect noticeable improvement. Conversely, if you have been on a medication for over 2 months and there is no evidence of improvement, it is quite probable that longer duration of treatment is not going to make a difference. Again, this is something that you should not decide by yourself; involve your healthcare provider.

Even a "Good" Prescription Medication Can Be Ineffective or Cause Adverse Effects

There are a number of different reasons why a well-indicated or appropriate prescription medication can be ineffective or result in adverse effects. Examples include:

- Medication-medication interactions: Maybe your provider did not know you were taking an interacting medication or supplement, or maybe you started an interacting medication sometime after prescription of the medication for your digestive problem.
- Pharmacogenomic factors: Your genetics may make a drug more or less effective, or more or less safe, etc.
- Dietary interactions: Eating certain foods may make a medication work more or less.
- Known adverse effects: Many prescription medications can cause constipation, diarrhea, or nausea in a significant proportion of patients. You might need an alternative medication, a lower dose, or something additional to manage an adverse effect.

Keep in mind the possibility of changes in your digestive problem as well. Some problems can become more severe over time, requiring more or stronger treatment. You could also have developed additional health conditions; perhaps the abdominal pain you are experiencing is not actually your colon this time but instead something wrong with your bladder that is mimicking colonic pain. All of this highlights the importance of vigilance, keeping an open mind, listening to your body, and communicating with your healthcare provider.

Duration of Treatment

How long you will need a medication will depend on the nature of your digestive problem. Duration may be short-term or long-term depending on your particular problem. Let us say you have a chronic digestive problem, like IBD, that requires continuous long-term treatment, but you autonomously decide to stop taking your medication because you are feeling well. If the problem comes back, you should not be surprised or feel let down by the medication or your healthcare provider. Rather, recognize that there was a mismatch in expectations; you have a chronic problem, and chronic problems typically require chronic treatment. On the other hand, say you used to have a lot of constipation or bloating a couple years ago for which you were put on a prescription medication, but since that time you have made important lifestyle and dietary modifications. It is quite possible that if you stop the prescription medication, you will do just fine—more exercise, losing excess weight, and incorporating more fiber in your diet may have been sufficient for you to maintain regular bowel habits. Because each scenario is unique, your expectations for the duration of treatment should be formulated together with your healthcare provider and tailored to your digestive problem.

The Optimal Long-Term Dose

With some digestive problems, once you are able to get the problem under control, you no longer need as much medication to *keep* it under control. That is to say, the maintenance dose may not need to be as high as the starting or "induction" dose. Enter here the notion of being on the "lowest effective dose of a medication", an important concept that I like to emphasize. Though not all medications have a good option for dose reduction, many if not most do. The lower the dose you are able to take while adequately maintaining control of your problem, the lower the likelihood of medication-related adverse effects. Lowering the dose of a medication is generally best done in conjunction with a healthcare provider, and a plan should be outlined as to how to go about it. While following the plan, you should be on the lookout for the possibility of your problem creeping back, or "recrudescence", which typically indicates a need to go back to a higher dose.

When/Whether to Consider Switching

Say you have a chronic digestive problem for which you have been taking a prescription medication for many months or even years, and for whatever reason you now wonder if you can switch to a different formulation, a newer version, or some completely different medication. This is a valid question. I tend to be a bit wary of medication switches in the absence of a compelling reason. That said, medicine is a dynamic field, and sometimes a switch does make good sense, especially if it is expected to make treatment safer, more effective, more convenient, and/or more affordable. These are important considerations that should be discussed with your healthcare provider to engage in shared decision-making.

Putting it all Together

OTC and prescription medications are essential for managing a wide variety of digestive problems. The options in this regard are practically innumerable and potentially overwhelming. There are certain advantages and disadvantages to both OTC and prescription medications which need to be considered depending on the clinical scenario. The use of these medications should be thoughtful and follow a number of fundamental principles that apply to digestive (as well as other health) problems, as was covered herein. Such an approach, together with appropriate involvement of a healthcare provider, is most likely to result in a favorable clinical outcome for one's health problem. Still, there are patients who prefer or need yet a different mode of treatment. Next, in Chap. 14, we review the role of complementary and alternative medicine in the management of digestive problems.

Further Reading

Alcoholic disease: liver and beyond. PubMed (nih.gov).
Behavioral gastroenterology: an emerging system and new frontier of action. PubMed (nih.gov).
Decreased sleep associated with constipation among U.S adults (healio.com).
Diet & lifestyle changes. About GERD.
Dietary fiber and the risk of acute diverticulitis. PubMed (nih.gov).
Disturbed sleep and disturbed bowel functions: implications for constipation in healthy individuals. PubMed (nih.gov).
Lifestyle changes. About Kids GI.
Lifestyle changes for gastroesophageal reflux disease. NYU Langone Health.
Sleep disturbances are linked to both upper and lower gastrointestinal symptoms in the general population. PubMed (nih.gov).
Smoking status and prevalence of upper gastrointestinal disorders. PubMed (nih.gov).

Chapter 14
Complementary and Alternative Medicine Approaches

What Is "CAM"?

It can be challenging to come up with a clear definition of the expression "complementary and alternative medicine". For practical purposes, I believe it can be defined as the collection of products and practices that are not part of conventional Western medicine. This is in keeping with the definition provided by the National Center for Complementary and Integrative Health (NCCIH), which classifies CAM therapies into two major subgroups:

1. Natural products: these include substances that are used to help strengthen and heal the body, such as herbal supplements, vitamins, and probiotics, among others.
2. Mind-body medicine practices: these include techniques and methods administered by a practitioner or performed independently by the patient, such as yoga, meditation, and biofeedback, among others (Table 14.1).

I will discuss each of these two subgroups further in this chapter. But first, let us touch upon some potential terminology issues with the expression "CAM".

Confusion Regarding the Expression "CAM"

There are many relevant and related terms that may be used in the context of "CAM", including alternative medicine, complementary medicine, functional medicine, integrative medicine, holistic medicine, natural medicine, traditional medicine, and others. These terms are frequently used interchangeably but may have subtle or even substantial differences depending on the context. Adding confusion to this is the fact that terminology has shifted over time. For example, the branch within the United States National Institutes of Health which studies CAM, presently

© The Author(s), under exclusive license to Springer Nature
Switzerland AG 2023
J. H. Tabibian, *Digestive Problems Solved*,
https://doi.org/10.1007/978-3-031-16317-3_14

Table 14.1 Mind-body medicine therapies encompassed in complementary and alternative medicine

Therapy	Overview of what it is
Acupuncture	A practice that involves pricking the skin with needles in targeted locations to restore qi, the vital life force that flows through the body, to alleviate pain and treat various physical, mental, and emotional conditions.
Anthroposophic medicine	Founded on the spiritual science of anthroposophy, a multimodal treatment based on the relationship between humans and nature which includes homeopathic and herbal medicine, art therapy, and rhythmical massage.
Ayurveda	The traditional Hindu system of holistic medicine based on the idea of balance in bodily systems through diet, herbal treatment, and yogic breathing.
Biofeedback	A process whereby electronic monitoring of a normally automatic body function is used to retrain an individual to acquire voluntary control over that function and leveraged to improve physical and mental health.
Cognitive behavioral therapy	A type of psychotherapy in which negative patterns of thought about the self, one's problems, and the world are challenged in order to alter unwanted behavior patterns, treat mood disorders, and better manage problems.
Homeopathy	A form of medicine based on the principle that "like should be cured with like" wherein disease is treated by minute doses of natural substances that in a healthy person would produce symptoms of disease.
Hypnosis	The induction of a deeply relaxed yet heightened focus state during which therapeutic suggestions are made to positively alter behavior and enhance relief of symptoms.
Meditation	A process of reflection and contemplation that allows an individual to focus thoughts, achieve mental clarity, and train attention to help alleviate symptoms.
Naturopathy	A system of medicine focusing on disease prevention and treatment through natural substances and methods that help the body heal itself.
Pilates	A system of exercise whereby controlled movements improve flexibility, build strength, develop endurance, and enhance mental awareness.
Qi Gong	A system of coordinated slow-flowing body movement, deep breathing, and meditation and breathing control related to tai chi, used for health, spirituality, and martial art.
Reiki	A healing technique based on the principle that a practitioner, using the power of touch, can channel energy into a patient to active natural healing processes and restore physical and mental wellbeing.
Relaxation practices	Techniques, such as diaphragmatic breathing, aimed to decrease tension and stress, control pain, and achieve other goals through activation of the parasympathetic nervous system.
Tai Chi	A Chinese philosophical concept and internal martial art which has evolved over the years and is practiced in the form of slow, controlled movements for defense training, health benefits, and meditation.
Traditional Chinese medicine	An ancient practice which brings the vital force of life, qi, into balance by affecting the complementary and opposing forces of qi, yin and yang.
Yoga	A philosophy and practice which includes physical postures, breathing techniques, and meditation to attain liberation from mind, body, and will and thereby promote physical and emotional Well-being.

Provided here is a high-level view of mind-body medicine forms. The list of therapies is not exhaustive and there may be overlap between therapies as well as variations within; other examples would include aromatherapy, electromagnetic therapy, chiropractic medicine, and massage therapy.

named the NCCIH, was originally established as the "Office of Alternative Medicine" and then renamed as the "National Center for Complementary and Alternative Medicine" before obtaining its present name. Another potential source of confusion is that while people often use "alternative" and "complementary" interchangeably, the two terms actually refer to different concepts, as follows:

- If a non-mainstream therapy, whether a natural product or a mind-body medicine technique, is used **together with** conventional medicine, it is considered "complementary."
- If a non-mainstream approach is used **instead of** conventional medicine, it is considered "alternative."

In other words, a non-mainstream approach such as an herbal supplement or meditation can be either complementary or alternative, depending on whether it is used together with or instead of conventional medical treatment.

When Can CAM Be Used?

While CAM has been most used and best studied in a small handful of common digestive problems, such as nausea, irritable bowel syndrome, dyspepsia, and constipation, it can be potentially helpful for many digestive problems, including organic GI disorders. As mentioned earlier, CAM can be classified into two subgroups—natural products and mind-body medicine practices. Within each of these there are an immense number of different forms, i.e. options. For almost any digestive problem, there is ostensibly at least one form of CAM that can improve one's quality of life, whether it is through effectuating less stress, less pain, or less anxiety. Though I practice conventional Western medicine, I see benefits in being inclusive and open-minded and not restricting a patient to conventional approaches. I welcome the complementary approach, especially for those in whom I think it can be of particular benefit. Why not try to leverage the best of both non-mainstream and conventional medicine, and accordingly tailor treatment to the individual and their digestive problem?

It is important to recognize that CAM is a treatment, and like treatments in conventional medicine, it is not always effective and may also have adverse effects. For instance, if you have a herniated disc in your back, yoga or Pilates may not be a good idea, or they may need to be modified to not worsen your back problem. Or if you are on blood thinners and/or planning to undergo surgery, certain herbal supplements can make your blood too thin. Therefore, I encourage patients to share their use of CAM with their healthcare providers so that informed, safe decisions can be made together. Admittedly, some providers see the use of CAM with cynicism, but it is better to let them know and be safe rather than keep it a secret and then be sorry. If the cynicism is excessive, perhaps a different, more flexible provider is needed. At the end of the day, there is no one-size-fits-all option, so CAM treatment should be individualized to the patient's needs, as with conventional treatment.

The First Subgroup of CAM: Natural Products

Natural products in the context of CAM come in a myriad of forms. What exactly natural products do and do not include can be difficult to define, but I tend to categorize them into:

- Botanicals or herbals
- vitamins/minerals
- probiotics
- miscellaneous supplements

Some might use the term "nutraceuticals" instead of "natural products" to distinguish these substances from "pharmaceuticals" used in conventional medicine, and that is okay. Whether you use the expression "natural products" or "nutraceuticals", recognize that these represent a massive industry occupying an immense amount of shelf space in pharmacies, supermarkets, and supplement stores, and totaling many billions of dollars spent per year in the United States alone. While many natural products are consumed by mouth as a pill, powder, or beverage, non-oral formulations exist as well, though they are typically not for digestive problems.

With so many natural product forms and options, it would be beyond the scope of this chapter to go into each one. I will instead provide some general principles regarding natural products as well as a primer on probiotics. For more information, I recommend the NCCIH website, which has a list of no less than 40 botanical products with accompanying summary profiles, as well as a section on vitamins and minerals with succinct yet handy information.

Things to Bear in Mind Regarding Natural Products

As can be seen on the NCCIH website, the amount of scientific evidence on natural products varies widely—there is a lot of information on some and extremely little on others. With natural products being used for so many different conditions, even if a given product has been "extensively" studied, it does not mean that it has been studied in a patient like you or for your digestive problem. Thus, it is important to be an informed consumer and maintain a degree of skepticism. If you are considering using a natural product, reflect on the possibility that it:

- may differ in important ways from the product tested in research studies, including concentration, total dose, preservatives, carriers, other additives, and type of encapsulation. Similarly, there are almost certainly differences between brands and maybe even between batches of a given brand. This heterogeneity introduces uncertainty and the possibility of variable results.
- could contains more than what is listed on the label. For example, some products marketed for weight loss, sexual enhancement, or bodybuilding have been found

to contain prescription drugs or other ingredients, some of which may be unsafe. I have actually encountered a few cases of liver failure associated with the use of such products.

- does not follow the same rules for manufacturing and distributing as conventional over-the-counter (OTC) or prescription medications. The process is more lax and less regulated, which usually gives me some pause and reason to ask the question "do I really need this product?"
- may interact with your medications or pose risks if you have certain medical conditions. Just because it is a natural product does not mean that it can't harm your body/GI system, though the risk overall is admittedly low. Still, you would hate to be that one person who sustains harm, especially from a product that you really did not need or that you could have known to avoid had you spoken to your healthcare provider.
- has probably not been tested in women who intend to become pregnant, are pregnant, or are nursing. These are probably not good scenarios in which to start a natural product.
- may not be enough to adequately treat your digestive problem. Even if you feel better when taking a natural product, it just may not be enough, as can be the case with conventional OTC or even prescription medications (see Chap. 13).
- is not always better to have more of a good thing. Taking more than the daily recommended dose of vitamins and minerals such as vitamin A, copper, iron, and zinc can throw the body off-balance. For instance, it can interfere with absorption of other vitamins and minerals and has been associated with various health hazards. Again, ask yourself, "do I really need this product?"

For the reasons outlined above, I do not widely recommend natural products to patients as a first or blanket measure. Instead, I evaluate the role and utility of a natural product on a case-by-case basis. For instance, sometimes a patient will continue to have symptoms despite appropriate conventional treatment of a digestive problem for which natural products have been well-studied. This is someone in whom I would welcome the opportunity to try the natural products that have been found to be effective and safe. Other times, patients will come to me already taking a natural product, and I will try to objectively review the pros, cons, and alternatives with them just as I would if they were on a conventional OTC or prescription medication. In some cases it makes sense to continue the product, but in others there will be really no appreciable benefit, and continued use is essentially a waste of time and money.

All in all, I encourage patients to use critical thinking coupled with a healthy dose of caution, in keeping with the central principle of medicine: "first, do no harm." Be careful to not be over-influenced by hype or marketing. Scrutinize it just as you would a conventional medicine, and do not ride naively on wishful thinking or a placebo effect while the digestive problem continues to affect your body. Lastly, be accepting of the possibility that you may need a conventional medicine or some other intervention in addition to or instead of a natural product.

A Primer on Probiotics

One of the most rapidly evolving forms of natural products, and perhaps the most fitting to be commented on by a gastroenterologist, is probiotics. Probiotics are microorganisms, mainly bacteria, which are beneficial to humans. You can think of probiotics as helping our digestive tract by crowding out any potentially bad microorganisms and using up nutrients that the bad microorganisms would need to propagate. However, how they actually work at a cellular and molecular level is much more complex and incompletely understood. Probiotics are available OTC and come in a variety of forms such as capsules, packets, and food products. The best-studied probiotic microorganisms are *Lactobacillus* and *Bifidobacterium*, both bacteria, and *Saccharomyces*, a yeast. The probiotics and brands I have seen used most in the clinic are:

- Visbiome® (formerly VSL#3®): a family of products centered around a probiotic mixture consisting of eight bacterial strains: Four strains of *Lactobacillus*, three strains of *Bifidobacterium, and one strain of Streptococcus. Available also as extra strength by prescription only.*
- Align®: a family of products centered around the patented probiotic bacterial strain *Bifidobacterium longum* 35,624™. Some products also contain "prebiotics", or compounds in food that increase probiotic growth and activity. The combination of prebiotics and probiotics is known as "synbiotics".
- Florastor®: a family of products centered around the yeast *Saccharomyces boulardii* CNCM I-745.

Yogurts such as Activia, Culturelle, and DanActive are also commonly used in clinic. However, regardless of the brand and the excitement over probiotics, going out and buying probiotics is not something that everyone needs to do. After all, how do you know what microorganism your intestinal microbiome is lacking or which microorganisms will do your GI system good? As discussed in Chap. 6, the microbiome, and by extension the use of probiotics as a therapy, is a field that is still very much in its infancy. We still have a lot to understand about the microorganisms within us, health, and disease, thus I would say it is good to use restraint.

Informed Use of Probiotics

So what digestive problems can probiotics be used for, and in whom? An ever-growing number of studies of specific probiotic species have suggested potential efficacy in a handful of digestive problems, the most studied of which are inflammatory bowel disease (particularly pouchitis and ulcerative colitis), antibiotic-related diarrhea, some forms of infectious diarrhea, irritable bowel syndrome, functional constipation, and hepatic encephalopathy. Yet probiotics do not have a role in every case, and their use should be guided by a healthcare provider on a case-by-case basis. Moreover, if you are using probiotics for a digestive problem not listed here, this should give you pause. There are many instances where probiotics are not doing much other than costing you time and money, or worse, potentially posing harm, as in immunosuppressed individuals.

Several societal practice guidelines and other references provided in the Further Reading section at the end of this chapter discuss when to consider the use of which probiotics in an evidence-based manner. I use these references to help inform and guide my decision-making and recommendations with regard to the use of probiotics. Notably, when suggesting probiotics, I do not lose sight of common household foods like yogurt as a source of probiotics—you do not always have to reach for an expensive capsule or a fancy brand. Lastly, I make individualized recommendations based on the patient and the digestive problem, as I do for non-probiotic natural products. Along these lines, I also avoid arguing with what works; that is, if a patient is taking a probiotic and it provides relief of a problem, I do not insist on stopping the probiotic simply because the textbook does not suggest it, especially if objective markers such as blood tests and/or scans are improving.

The Second Subgroup of cam: Mind-Body Medicine

Mind-body medicine is the second of two major subgroups of CAM. It comes in numerous forms, some more common and easier to find than others (Table 14.1). There can also be different types of a given form of mind-body medicine, such as acupuncture and electroacupuncture, as well as variation between practitioners in their personal styles, philosophies, and preferred maneuvers and techniques. Not all options or practitioners will be a good fit for a given individual or problem. Some trial and error is often needed to find what works, depending on the available options as well as personal priorities and the problem at hand. Input from a healthcare provider can be useful to help assess options and guide the way. As mentioned earlier, though, some providers are less open than others to such discussion or may have very limited knowledge about mind-body medicine, especially forms that are relatively esoteric.

Mind-body medicine may not cure digestive problems, especially organic GI disorders, but it can certainly improve quality of life as well as associated anxiety, depression, pain, and stress. The major downsides with mind-body medicine, aside from the fact that not all forms have been studied specifically for managing digestive problems, are that they can be costly, often not covered by insurance, and time-consuming. Finding the money and time for it can be challenging for many, though I will say that setting time aside for one's health and wellness is exactly what many people with digestive problems need. As challenging as it was to arrange, I recall how helpful it was for me to have time set aside for acupuncture when I was experiencing a health problem a number of years ago. While acupuncture alone was not enough for me, it did help in a complementary fashion to conventional Western medicine, in addition to giving me more perspective as a patient.

Since entire books can be written on just a single form of mind-body medicine, I will not attempt to specifically discuss all the different forms of mind-body medicine aside from the information in Table 14.1. However, I will discuss those that comprise what is known as "behavioral therapy".

Behavioral Therapy

Behavioral therapy is an umbrella term for a broad range of techniques that look to identify and help change maladaptive behaviors while also reinforcing healthy behaviors. I am making a special mention of behavioral therapy for five reasons. First, it is particularly well-studied, including but not limited to its role in managing digestive problems. Second, it is typically more likely to be covered by insurance as compared to most other forms of mind-body medicine. Third, there are GI psychologists and other dedicated professionals who specialize in behavioral therapy focused on managing GI problems; they use behavioral treatments to leverage and positively influence the interconnected relationship between digestive and emotional health as part of a whole-person approach to wellness. Fourth, it is extremely safe for the vast majority of patients. Lastly, if there is a stigma associated with receiving behavioral therapy, I would like to de-stigmatize it. You do not have to have a mental illness to receive behavioral therapy, nor does receiving it mean that you are "crazy" and that there is not merit to your digestive problem. You may be a good candidate for behavioral therapy if any of the following apply:

- You find that life stressors make your digestive problem worse.
- You are excessively worried about the impact of your digestive problem.
- You have trouble relaxing, in general or because you're fixated on your digestive problem.
- You are experiencing anxiety or depression because of your digestive problem.
- You perceive or are told that you are exhausting pharmacological options.

There are several types of behavioral therapy applicable to digestive problems, including but not limited cognitive behavioral therapy (CBT), biofeedback, stress management therapy, and gut-directed hypnotherapy. Let us take a high-level look at the first three, which are the most proven for digestive problems.

Cognitive Behavioral Therapy

CBT is the most thoroughly researched behavioral therapy form available and has been studied in the context of a wide number of digestive problems. The premise of CBT and its various forms is based on the "five areas" model, as shown in Fig. 14.1. This model holds that our experience with a situation, for instance a digestive problem, is based on its interaction with our environment, which includes both our

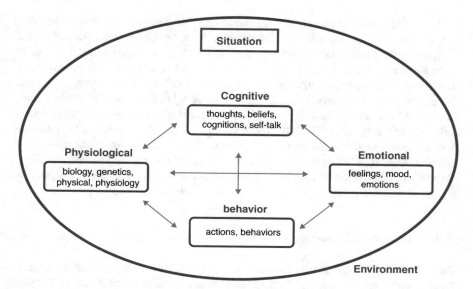

Fig. 14.1 According to the "five areas" cognitive behavioral therapy model, our experience with a situation is defined by the interactions between our environment and four interlinked factors: cognitive, emotional, physiological, and behavioral

present setting as well as the past (e.g. family history and previous relationships), and four interlinked areas or factors, namely:

- thoughts/cognitions
- emotions
- physiology/symptoms
- behaviors

The cognitive model holds that the way an individual perceives and experiences a situation is more closely connected to their reaction to the situation rather than the situation itself. I do not necessarily think this is true with all situations, but I definitely do think our reaction to a situation plays an important role in how it impacts us. CBT helps make sense of what often seems like an overwhelming problem by breaking it down into smaller parts and seeing how the five areas above may influence each other and aggravate the problem. During CBT, a GI psychologist or therapist works with a patient to uncover how they think about themselves, their problems, others, and the world, and to identify which thoughts are helpful and which are not. The duo work together to interrupt and change unhelpful thinking patterns which subsequently give rise to negative emotions, behaviors, and symptoms. As the thinking patterns change, so do the aforementioned four interlinked areas, thereby bringing about relief. CBT is a structured intervention, focused on addressing specific problems and designed to take place over a limited amount of time, with the majority of patients gaining the most benefit within ten sessions.

To provide an example of an application of CBT, imagine a young, otherwise healthy patient who experiences intermittent bloating discomfort. An unhelpful thinking pattern would be for the patient to believe this is a sign of a stomach ulcer or an issue with the pancreas based on commercials he has seen. This thinking can then spiral into negative emotions and depressed mood, excess worrying, and even feeling fatigued and weak. Interrupting this thinking pattern and the ensuing cascade of effects, for instance by recognizing that the bloating most likely is just a reflection of eating high FODMAP foods (Chap. 12) and their resultant gas production, can undo much of the negative experience that occurs in association with the bloating. Overall, CBT is a cornerstone of behavioral therapy and something that I have recommended to and observed be beneficial for numerous patients with digestive problems, including functional as well as organic GI disorders.

Stress Management Therapy

There are various forms of stress management therapy. Talk therapy and instruction in simple techniques such as diaphragmatic breathing, relaxation training, and resilience-building methods are among some of the forms. Through any one of these, patients are helped to identify tools they can rely on to keep stress in check, including stress which arises from digestive problems. Of these various forms of stress management therapy, I am most familiar with diaphragmatic breathing and can attest to its efficacy based on what I have observed. Diaphragmatic breathing facilitates the activation of the parasympathetic nervous system, which can be thought of as the relaxation response of the body or the "rest and digest", non- "fight or flight" state. I have seen diaphragmatic breathing work wonders for patients with rumination syndrome, fecal urgency, and constipation, among other problems. As with other forms of stress management therapy, it is as safe as a treatment can be, portable, and widely applicable.

Biofeedback Therapy

Biofeedback is a behavioral intervention that can be used to learn to better control your body's functions, such as your heart rate. During biofeedback therapy, you are connected to electrical sensors that help you receive information, or "feedback", about your body. This feedback helps you proactively make changes in your body, such as relaxing or contracting certain muscles, to achieve the results you want, whether it is reducing pain, evacuating your bowels, or holding stool back to avoid incontinence. In essence, biofeedback gives you the ability to practice new ways to actively control certain body functions and increase awareness of bodily cues. There are numerous types of biofeedback, as well as different biofeedback devices. The applications of biofeedback are broad and include digestive problems such as constipation, fecal incontinence, irritable bowel syndrome, and chronic pain, in addition to numerous other physical and mental health issues. As with diaphragmatic breathing, I have seen biofeedback work wonders. Finding the right practitioner or therapist can be challenging, and it does require a fair amount of effort on the part of the patient, but it often pays off.

Integrative Medicine: Taking cam to the Next Level

As a closing thought, I believe it is worth mentioning "integrative medicine" or "integrative health", which in some ways represents an evolution and the most progressive application of CAM. It is a combination approach which brings conventional and complementary approaches together in a coordinated manner, as illustrated in Fig. 14.2. Integrative medicine embraces multimodal interventions such as conventional medicine, lifestyle and dietary changes, CAM, and other approaches in various combinations, with an emphasis on treating the person as a whole rather than one organ system or an isolated problem. This form of coordinate care is a lofty aim in the fast-paced way healthcare is currently delivered, if nothing else because it poses various logistical challenges. However, I think it has the potential of offering the best possible treatment options and outcomes for patients and their digestive problems. Whereas CAM has historically been conceptualized as being effective for mainly functional rather than organic GI disorders, I believe integrative medicine can be quite effective for both.

Putting it all Together

Many patients will at some point try CAM in one form or another for the management of their digestive problems. CAM is based on a holistic, "non-mainstream" approach to treatment and encompasses a vast array of forms. The various forms of CAM can be categorized as either natural products or mind-body medicine practices. The former is a huge category which includes botanicals, vitamins/minerals, and probiotics, and this chapter has provided an overview and some pearls in this regard. The latter is also a large category (Table 14.1), with some forms of mind-body medicine practices being more evidence-based than others; the best studied is behavioral therapy such as CBT (Fig. 14.1). Despite generally being safe, some forms of CAM do carry risk, and some are costly without doing much if any good. For these reasons and others, CAM is not for every patient, and it should be used in a thoughtful, objective manner, with input from a healthcare professional whenever possible. Following an ideal integrative medicine approach (Fig. 14.2), CAM would be just one part of multimodal, coordinated care which brings different approaches together to best treat the patient as a whole.

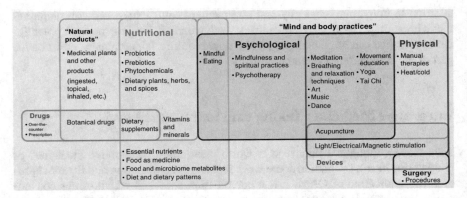

Fig. 14.2 An integrative medicine treatment approach grouped by psychological, physical, and nutritional categories. Adapted from Complementary, Alternative, or Integrative Health: What's In a Name? I NCCIH (nih.gov)

Further Reading

AGA clinical practice guidelines on the role of probiotics in the management of gastrointestinal disorders (gastrojournal.org).

Biofeedback. Mayo Clinic.

Complementary and alternative medicine for functional gastrointestinal disorders. PubMed (nih.gov).

Complementary, alternative, or integrative health: what's in a name? NCCIH (nih.gov).

Frontiers. A review of the effects of natural compounds, medicinal plants, and mushrooms on the gut microbiota in colitis and cancer. Pharmacology (frontiersin.org).

GI health psychology. Integrative Digestive Health and Wellness Program. Los Angeles, CA (ucla-health.org).

Nutraceuticals in gastrointestinal disorders. ScienceDirect.

Probiotics for gastrointestinal conditions: a summary of the evidence. American Family Physician (aafp.org).

Types of complementary and alternative medicine. Johns Hopkins Medicine.

World Gastroenterology Organisation practice guideline.

Correction to: Digestive Problems Solved

Correction to:
Chapter 2 and 8 in: J. H. Tabibian, *Digestive Problems Solved*,
https://doi.org/10.1007/978-3-031-16317-3

The original version of chapter 2 was published with an incorrect link in the Further Reading section (page 16), http://clevelandclinic.org/.

It has now been corrected to https://my.clevelandclinic.org/health/articles/7040-gastrointestinal-diseases.

The original version of chapter 8 was published with incorrect links in the Further Reading section (page 64), https://www.aafp.org/afp/2012/0201/afp20120201p279.pdf

https://www.acponline.org/system/fles/documents/clinical_information/high_value_care/clinician_resources/hvcc_toolkit/hvcc_project/generic-referral-to-subspecialist-practice.pdf

These links have now been corrected to https://www.aafp.org/pubs/afp/issues/2012/0201/p279.html

https://www.acponline.org/clinical-information/high-

The updated original version of this chapter can be found at
https://doi.org/10.1007/978-3-031-16317-3_2
https://doi.org/10.1007/978-3-031-16317-3_8

Index

© The Editor(s) (if applicable) and The Author(s), under exclusive license to
Springer Nature Switzerland AG 2023
J. H. Tabibian, *Digestive Problems Solved*,
https://doi.org/10.1007/978-3-031-16317-3

Printed in the United States
by Baker & Taylor Publisher Services